STORIES ARE WHAT SAVE US

STORIES ARE WHAT SAVE US

A Survivor's Guide to Writing about Trauma

DAVID CHRISINGER

Foreword by Brian Turner | Afterword by Angela Ricketts

JOHNS HOPKINS UNIVERSITY PRESS | *Baltimore*

Johns Hopkins University Press
2715 North Charles Street
Baltimore, Maryland 21218-4363
www.press.jhu.edu

Library of Congress Cataloging-in-Publication Data

Names: Chrisinger, David, 1986– author.
Title: Stories are what save us : a survivor's guide to writing about trauma /
    David Chrisinger ; foreword by Brian Turner ; afterword by Angela Ricketts.
Description: Baltimore : Johns Hopkins University Press, 2021. |
    Includes bibliographical references and index.
Identifiers: LCCN 2020030798 | ISBN 9781421440804 (paperback) |
    ISBN 9781421440811 (ebook)
Subjects: LCSH: Chrisinger, David, 1986—Mental health. | Post-traumatic stress disorder—
    Treatment—United States. | Psychic trauma—United States—Biography.
Classification: LCC RC552.P67 C475 2021 | DDC 616.85/21—dc23
LC record available at https://lccn.loc.gov/2020030798

A catalog record for this book is available from the British Library.

Special discounts are available for bulk purchases of this book. For more information, please contact Special Sales at specialsales@jh.edu.

Johns Hopkins University Press uses environmentally friendly book materials, including recycled text paper that is composed of at least 30 percent post-consumer waste, whenever possible.

Write. Find a way to keep alive and write. There is nothing else to

say . . . Talent is insignificant. I know a lot of talented ruins. Beyond

talent lie all the usual words: discipline, love, luck,

but most of all: ENDURANCE.

—*James Baldwin*

"The Art of Fiction No. 78," interview by Jordan Elgrably,

Paris Review

CONTENTS

BRIAN TURNER

Author of *My Life as a Foreign Country: A Memoir*

I write this message to you as a novel coronavirus (COVID-19) has reached and sustained pandemic levels. The entire medical system in the United States is scrambling to effectively battle the disease. Unemployment lines are growing desperately long, and an eviction crisis appears to be right around the corner. Many Americans not deemed essential workers are sheltering in place. It is a time of lockdowns and partial lockdowns and attempts to reopen the country in a manner that's safe and sound. It is a time of masks and respirators, social distancing, separation, isolation.

And throughout it all, I've been reading David Chrisinger's phenomenal new book, *Stories Are What Save Us*. I use the singular—book—but it would be more accurate to say that the volume you're about to read contains several books woven into one. It is, overall, a book-length braided tutorial on the process of writing one's story so that it might be shared with another. Part writing guidebook, part memoir, part teaching handbook—*Stories Are What Save Us* manages to reveal and to share writing lessons and life lessons all in one very readable volume.

A Writer's Guidebook

The relaxed and conversational approach that Chrisinger takes in this book removes the distance between author and student. But don't be fooled: This is a master class on writing done to a book-length scale. It's hands-on work, too, as Chrisinger rolls up his sleeves to dive into each sentence and paragraph in order to explore the inner architecture of the storyteller's medium. In this sense, the book itself serves as a kind of portable classroom—offering a wide range of craft tools and structures to aid in the framing and unfolding of your story. Part of what makes this book especially helpful is that Chrisinger manages to interweave his own process as a writer in order to model the techniques and approaches that will help you as you tell your own story.

A Memoir

There is a profoundly moving and compelling memoir threaded throughout this book. Most writers would be (rightfully) satisfied with having created such a layered and rich memoir—and they'd simply publish it on its own. As a stand-alone book, Chrisinger's memoir would be praised, and he would receive warranted attention from his peers for having written a meaningful and nuanced book, one worthy of a good reader's time. But Chrisinger is on a much larger, selfless mission here. With this book, he invites the reader to sit beside him as he writes his memoir—so that he might share his reasons for the choices made in crafting the story. But it isn't just the story that he's after. It's something much larger. He's done all of this so that we might begin to process the trauma and conflicts within ourselves by learning how to tell our own stories. In so doing, it's possible that we might become more whole in the process.

A Teacher's Handbook

While not overtly written as a handbook for educators, this book will surely aid teachers in a variety of ways. Its structure provides writing communities with a template for short-form intensive work, as well as a set of long-form modules spread over a semester or even an entire academic year, replete with supplemental appendix material.

As our country learns to adapt during this current pandemic, the issues involved in creating and nurturing deep and meaningful connections with one another have become more and more illuminated. Of course, these issues involved in connecting with one another are not new. For those who have experienced trauma and have struggled to articulate their complicated and layered experiences—all those messy and fragmented aspects of memory that come with being human—David Chrisinger has created this book for you. He knows that your story is important and that only you can tell it. He's here to help you do just that.

The time has come for me to step out of the way so that you and David can get to work drafting that story. So fire up your laptop, get your notebook ready, and turn to page 1.

It's time to start writing!

— —— —

Brian Turner is the author of the memoir *My Life as a Foreign Country* and two collections of poetry—*Here, Bullet* and *Phantom Noise*. His essays and poetry have been published in the *New York Times*, *National Geographic*, *Poetry Daily*, the *Georgia Review*, the *Virginia Quarterly Review*, and several other journals. He has received a USA Hillcrest Fellowship in Literature, a Literature Fellowship in Poetry from the National Endowment for the Arts, the Poets' Prize, and a fellowship from the Lannan Foundation. He earned an MFA from the University of Oregon before serving for seven years in the US Army. For a year in Iraq, Brian served as an infantry team leader with the 3rd Stryker Brigade Combat Team, 2nd Infantry Division. Prior to that, he deployed to Bosnia-Herzegovina with the 10th Mountain Division.

In addition to being an infantryman, poet, and memoirist, Brian has worked as a machinist, a locksmith's assistant, a convenience store clerk, a pickler, a maker of circuit boards, a dishwasher, a teacher of English as a foreign language in South Korea, a low-voltage electrician, a radio DJ, a bass guitar instructor, and more. He also directs the MFA program at Sierra Nevada College and serves as a contributing editor for the *Normal School*.

Before we begin, I would like to acknowledge the extraordinary debt I owe to the teachers, writers, and editors who have taught me such wise things about writing over the years: Brian Castner, Matthew J. Hefti, Benjamin Busch, Anna Hiatt, Alexis Clark, Jesse Goolsby, Lu-Ann Zieman, Mary Doyle, Liesel Kershul, Tracy Crow, Eric Chandler, Brian Turner, Kayla M. Williams, Peter Molin, Abby Murray, Jerri Bell, Angela Ricketts, Jenny Pacanowski, Drew Pearl, Teresa Fazio, Lauren Katzenberg, David Georgi, Dario DiBattista, Sue Petrie, Matthew Komatsu, David P. Ervin, Maureen Giblin, Matt Gallagher, Phil Klay, Sebastian Junger, Avi Sharma, Kevin Cullen, Karen Stabiner, Stuart Krichevsky, Andria Williams, and Jennifer Orth-Veillon.

The following essays originally appeared in other publications; all have been edited and revised for this collection. "I Grew Up Believing My Grandfather Was a War Hero" was first published by the *New York Times Magazine*. "Baggage," "When I Think about My Son," "Hold My Housing Until I'm OK," "Learning the Power of Connection and Companionship," "Losing the Fear That He Abandoned His Men," and "Trapped in the Amber of This Moment" originally appeared in The War Horse. *War, Literature & the Arts* published "In the Shadow of an Unanswered Question," and "If You Want to Travel Far, Go Together" appeared in *Retire the Colors*, published by Hudson Whitman/ Excelsior College Press. Lastly, "The Rules Do Not Apply" was published in *O-Dark-Thirty*, and "Everything Had Changed, and Nothing Was Different" first appeared in *Collateral Magazine*. It is my hope that presented together, and expanded upon, the sum of my work is greater than its parts.

Many thanks to the brilliant editors who helped me shape my prose and put the right words in the correct order: Anna Hiatt, Alexis Clark, and the entire team at The War Horse, Jesse Goolsby at *War, Literature & the Arts*, Lauren Katzenberg and David Georgi at the *New York Times Magazine*, Jerri Bell and Dario DiBattista at the Veterans Writing Project, and Abby Murray at *Collateral Magazine*.

I'd also like to thank the following people at the University of Wisconsin–Stevens Point and the nonprofit organizations the Veteran Print Project; Team Red, White & Blue; and The War Horse for their enthusiasm, kindness, and continued support: Nancy LoPattin-Lummis, Ann Whipp, Bob Erickson, Lee Willis, Valerie Barske, Yvette M. Pino, Jonathan Silk, Zack Armstrong, Joe Quinn, Sarah Roberts, Mike Greenwood, Blayne Smith, Thomas Brennan, John Edelman, and Lindsey Melki.

I would be remiss to point out that I simply would not be able to do what I do without the continual support, tireless effort, and incredible vision of my editor, Robin Coleman. Kudos are also due to Robert M. Brown, who copyedited this book with enormous skill and warmth and precision.

Lastly, I'd like to mention that without the love and understanding of my beautiful wife, Ashley, who selflessly puts up with my absences, shoulders the brunt of the workload raising our three children—George, Henry, and Stella—and continues to believe in me and my work, this book would not exist. As my first reader, Ashley regularly makes the value of my work visible to me in myriad ways and reaches for me whenever I stumble. Her love is the center of my world. I do not exaggerate when I say that I could not be who I am without her.

STORIES ARE WHAT SAVE US

Introduction

Atonement

B ELIEVE ME," he said as he reached into his back-right jeans pocket. "I know this is a big ask." With his left hand he was gripping two glass bottles of Pabst Blue Ribbon by their necks. His gaze was focused on the concrete floor in front of my workbench, one of the few spots in the garage that wasn't cluttered with precariously stacked cardboard boxes and bits of random furniture. My wife and I had recently bought a small home with good bones less than a block from the university where I was teaching a writing seminar for student veterans, and we hadn't even come close to finishing all the unpacking.

As he pulled his right hand from his pocket, I saw that he was holding something dark and metal looking, about the size of his palm. "I don't have anyone else," he said, handing me what I realized was the trigger housing for his M14 rifle. I had been able to recognize its look and feel so quickly only because I had visited a shooting range with him and another student of mine the weekend before. He had let me fire what he said was one of his most prized possessions. The other two were his dog, a black Lab named Duchess, and a glossy black Harley-Davidson motorcycle. I don't remember if the bike had a name.

"What do you want me to do with this?" I asked. I couldn't look him in the eye, so I stared at the round trigger housing. All I can remember in the moments after that question had left my mouth was the crackle of the fluorescent light hanging above my head suddenly becoming louder, then fading as my attention turned back to him.

"Just hold onto it for me for a while," he said. I lifted my gaze to meet his. "I don't trust myself with it right now."

That was back in the early months of 2015. I hadn't yet earned my various certifications in suicide prevention. I didn't know how to help someone who was thinking of hurting themselves. I didn't know the right questions to ask or how important it is not only to persuade them to seek help but also to hand them over, personally, to a qualified professional who can deliver that help.

My student who handed me his trigger housing never held me responsible for how he was feeling that night. But a couple of days after his visit, it became clear that I was at least partly to blame. A few hours before he asked if he could come over to talk, a Marine he had served with in Afghanistan, a man he had looked up to and had aspired to be like one day, had read an essay my student had written in my class, which I had edited and posted to our class's website. He told my student that everyone who knew him would be better off if he swallowed the barrel of a pistol.

— —— —

On the first day of class that semester, about a month before my student left the trigger housing with me for safekeeping, he arrived before most of the other students and sat in the second row. He was wearing a baggy flannel shirt and jeans and looked like a Seattle grunge rocker, minus the long hair. The fitted gray baseball cap he wore, along with his three-day-old blond chin scruff, made it hard to discern the angles of his facial features. As the other students shuffled in and jockeyed for seats in the back row or against the wall, he told me that he'd been thinking a lot about all these stories he had inside him and that he was excited finally to be in a class that would help him get them out.

Later that week, he told me that when he was in the Marines, he had found out he was headed to Afghanistan even before he finished his advanced training and reported to his unit. "I was freaking out the whole time," he explained to me in an interview I conducted with him as part of the Library of Congress's Veterans History Project. "My instructor had this graduation poster of everyone from a previous class," he said, miming as though he was holding a large poster with both hands above his head, "and one day everyone was fuckin' around. My instructor grabbed the poster and yelled at us, 'Hey, fuck faces, come here and look at this. You know what this is? This is my class from two cycles ago.' There were Xs over most of the faces." An X over the face was a crude way of showing which Marines had been killed or wounded in their first deployment in Afghanistan. "I can't wait until I get your fuckin' class's poster," he said, imitating the salty instructor, "and I can start crossing all your fuckin' faces off."

He paused. Then he lowered his arms. He looked like he was collecting his thoughts, like he was searching for the right words.

"I didn't deal with any of the shit that well," he said.

During the rest of the interview, he told me more about his fears and anxieties, about the psychological toll that IEDs (improvised explosive devices) take on a young man. He said he had seen enough guys lose legs in Afghanistan to know that if he had to be wounded, he'd prefer being shot to being blown up. At one point, his tone and demeanor changed. He sat up tall in his chair, his face deadly serious. "It's a privilege to be able to shoulder that burden and allow civilians at home to be ignorant of all the terrible shit in the world," he said, pausing for effect. "Ignorance is bliss, and it's a fucking privilege and an honor to carry that weight for them. That ignorance—of having to face your own mortality—is one of the greatest gifts we give to civilians."

— — —

Talking with my student about his experiences was exciting, intoxicating even. I learned much too late, however, that there is a fine line between intoxicating and painful, especially when stories like his are handled indelicately. Not knowing then what I know now, I urged him to write, even if his stories came out as garbage on the page—something many first-time writers fear. "All first drafts are shit," I told him reassuringly. "But that's why I'm here, to help you say what you need to say."

I am not a psychologist. In graduate school, I studied European history and social science theory, and when the Great Recession hit the academic job market in 2009, I jumped ship for a communications job in the federal government. For nearly a decade, I helped economists, statisticians, and public policy experts write program evaluations, governmental audits, and policy proposals for Congress, converting complex data into understandable narratives. The director who plucked my application from the slush pile said he had hired me, partly at least, because historians know how to tell good stories supported by evidence.

My work with military veterans didn't start until one of my childhood best friends, Brett Foley, returned from Afghanistan in 2010. After spending nine months in a combat zone and about as many months struggling with the aftereffects, he confided in me that he needed help. Not knowing what else I could do to support him, I encouraged Brett to write about what he had experienced during his years in the Marine Corps. It took a few weeks of coaxing, but eventually Brett took my advice, and he started typing out memories, everything from funny anecdotes from boot camp to stories of the most traumatic moments of his life. When he had written all he thought he could, he would send me his words. My first instinct was always to try to edit, but instead I would ask him questions about what he had written to help him fill in the missing details.

As Brett was writing his stories and responding to my questions, I read everything I could get my hands on that might help me better understand what he was going through. The first gold mine I stumbled upon was *Trauma and Recovery* by Dr. Judith Lewis Herman. "The conflict between the will to deny horrible events and the will to proclaim them aloud," she writes in the introduction, "is the central dialectic of psychological trauma. People who have survived atrocities often tell their stories in a highly emotional, contradictory, and fragmented manner which undermines their credibility, and thereby serves the twin imperatives of truth-telling and secrecy. When the truth is finally recognized, survivors can begin their recovery."[1]

After months of my helping pull out and shape stories from Brett's past, he and his wife, Whitney, found themselves in a place where it was possible to begin putting back together the pieces of their lives that had been shattered by war. They bought a house. Brett enrolled in a criminal justice program at a technical college. He quit drinking himself to sleep each night, was better able to control his temper, had more energy, and started feeling more comfortable in crowds, too. Most importantly, Brett and Whitney started holding space for each other, listening to what the other needed, despite all that still needed to be resolved.

At the time, I wasn't aware that what I had done, essentially, was guide Brett through an extended "expressive writing" exercise, nor did I know anything about all the research that has gone into this type of therapeutic intervention.[2] All I knew then was that writing about his traumatic experiences seemed to be what had helped my friend more than anything else he had tried.

In the fall of 2013, I proposed a writing course exclusively for student veterans to a state school in Wisconsin. The curriculum I designed was based entirely on what I had done informally with Brett after he returned from Afghanistan. With all the confidence of an expert unencumbered by much experience, I convinced the school's administrators that providing a classroom space where veterans would have the opportunity to write about trauma and share those stories with empathetic readers could be the start of something transformative.

—— —— ——

The student who had given me his trigger housing that night in my garage turned in a short essay a few days after I interviewed him for the Veterans History Project. Raw and unpolished, it detailed a recurring nightmare that plagued him most nights and tormented him in his waking hours as well. I found it deeply confessional and achingly sincere, though it wasn't a coherent tale in the style most readers would likely appreciate. It was more like a superstructure of immersive fragments and detailed streams of consciousness. Still, there was something impressive about it, and I thought that, with a little editing, his story would be ready to post on our class's website.

Shortly after I posted his essay, my student shared a link to it on his Facebook page. He tagged his friends, family members, and other young men he'd served with as if to say, "Read this. It will explain everything." Within a few hours, dozens of positive comments stacked up like dinner plates below his post. I wasn't the only reader who had been sucked into the harrowing and intimate nature of his story.

Before too long, however, the comments being left by readers turned sour. It began with a threatening message from a Marine, the one he had once looked up to, who thought my student was blowing his trauma out of proportion. My student's deployment had been cake, according to this other Marine, which apparently meant my student had no right to claim he had suffered any kind of psychological wounds. For the next couple of days, this Marine tagged dozens of other Marines who chimed in to question my student's account and to harass him on deeply personal levels.

After deleting his original post, along with all the positive comments his story initially received, my student texted me that he needed to talk. That was the same night he asked me to hold onto his trigger housing. Once I learned what my student had experienced because of the essay he wrote, I felt a sludge build in my stomach, a pressure behind my eyes. I felt eaten raw, simultaneously responsible and insignificant and irredeemable. An editor's job, as I view it now, is not simply to correct comma splices and other grammatical errors but also to humbly enter a writer's story and help prune what isn't needed and transplant what's needed to strengthen it.

But I didn't do that.

I should have pushed him to reveal what he had learned, how he had changed, and in what ways he had grown. I should have coached him to present his own truth, not to persuade readers, but rather to gently challenge readers to draw their own conclusions.

But I didn't.

— — —

A few days later, I reread my student's essay. A new feeling came over me. I was shivering without being cold. And the shivering wouldn't stop. So I stopped. I had to. Sitting cross-legged on the floor at the foot of my bed, I wrapped a blanket around my drooping shoulders to stave off the chill. My wife was running errands with our two young boys, and there was no one else in the house I could talk things through with. Then I remembered something. In a cardboard box at the bottom of my closet I had a small paperback copy of a book I often turned to in times of great doubt or despair: Viktor Frankl's *Man's Search for Meaning*.

First published in 1946, the book recounts Frankl's journey of survival through several Nazi concentration camps during World War II. Dog-eared and heavily marked up, the pages in my copy were yellowing and felt brittle to my touch. I gently flipped page after page, looking for a passage I knew I had underlined during one of the several times I had read the book cover to cover. I found what I was searching for: "A man's suffering is similar to the behavior of gas," Frankl says. "If a certain quantity of gas is pumped into an empty chamber, it will fill the chamber completely and evenly, no matter how big the chamber. Thus suffering completely fills the human soul and conscious mind, no matter whether the suffering is great or little." Therefore, Frankl concludes, "the 'size' of human suffering is absolutely relative."[3]

My student's story wasn't that he went to war, suffered, survived, came home, and struggled with a debilitating nightmare. That's just the plot. After multiple rounds of editing and revision, my student discovered that what he was truly struggling with was the fear and guilt associated with feeling traumatized despite not having experienced the level of trauma others around him had survived. Uncovering that story and writing to it—rather than away from it—helped him confront his fears and painful memories, which robbed them of their power. By understanding what his story was really about, my student was able to name his emotions and find a way to view his trauma from a different perspective, which helped him begin to resolve it. He didn't push his pain away or endlessly ruminate over what happened. He didn't try to reframe it and pretend that what he had survived was good for him. Instead, he found coherence and meaning in the construction of a story that transcended the limits of his personal tragedy. And with a little coaching on finding the story *underneath* his story, the final draft of his essay, which was subsequently included in a collection I edited that was published a year later,[4] flowed directly from how he made sense of what he had experienced in Afghanistan and how he measured what mattered most to him.

"I remember two cases of would-be suicide," Frankl writes later on in *Man's Search for Meaning*. "Both men had talked of their intentions to commit suicide. Both used the typical argument—they had nothing more to expect from life. In both cases it was a question of getting them to realize that life was still expecting something from them; something in the future was expected of them."[5]

"A man who becomes conscious of the responsibility he bears toward a human being," Frankl continues, "or to an unfinished work, will never be able to throw away his life. He knows the 'why' for his existence, and will be able to bear almost any 'how.'"[6]

— — —

This book is my attempt at atonement for my past sin of exploitation. I didn't know back when my student wrote the first draft of his essay how difficult it is to negotiate matters of identity and adversity in front of an anonymous crowd of online readers ready to shame and distance themselves from personal storytellers. I know now, and in the intervening years since I published that student's essay, I have learned much about how to tell a personal story about trauma that leads to connection and understanding. This book, in short, details what I've learned along the way. It is my hope that the principles and guidance contained here will help you avoid the trial-and-error approach to writing, which I had to take, by giving you the tools you need to home in on a story and begin writing with confidence.

— — —

But what if you're not a combat veteran? It doesn't matter. Trauma is trauma, as Frankl would say. Most of us have survived some form of it in our lifetime. In 2013, research led by Dean G. Kilpatrick indicated that rates of trauma among American adults might be far higher than had previously been assumed. Specifically, Kilpatrick's research team found that nearly 90 percent of people they studied reported having been exposed to at least one type of event deemed traumatic by the *Diagnostic and Statistical Manual of Mental Disorders*, fifth edition. Such events include those considered natural, or "acts of God": disasters, accidents, or fires. Other traumatic events sound industrial and are usually the result of circumstance: exposure to hazardous chemicals or harsh working conditions. Then there are the traumatic events of human design: combat or war zone exposure; physical or sexual assault; witnessing physical or sexual assault; unexpectedly seeing dead bodies or body parts; and threat to, injury, or death of a family member or close friend owing to violence.[7]

Even as I write these words, Americans across the country who have never set foot on a battlefield are, like me, sheltering in place because of the coronavirus pandemic. Uncertainty. Upheaval. Unemployment. Illness and death. Depending on who you are and what you've already survived, the pandemic may be a frightening and anxiety-inducing disruption to the status quo—or it may be downright traumatic. We know from previous research on the Ebola virus that medical professionals and those directly impacted by the virus are particularly susceptible to experiencing anxiety and depression and developing post-traumatic stress disorder.[8]

With all that in mind, I think Judith Herman sums up nicely what it means to experience trauma. "Unlike commonplace misfortunes," she writes, "traumatic events generally involve threats to life or bodily integrity, or a close personal encounter with violence and death. They confront human beings with the extremities of helplessness and terror, and evoke the response of catastrophe."[9] The collection of student essays I edited is a perfect example of this. There are, of course, stories of combat trauma included in the collection. But there are also stories of sifting through the rubble and scraps of human remains at the Pentagon in the days after the terrorist attacks of September 11, 2001, and in Japan after the Fukushima nuclear disaster 10 years later. There are also stories of undiagnosed and mysterious physical ailments and the pain of being ostracized by friends and family who struggled to understand experiences unlike their own. Trauma is trauma. Viewed through a less clinical and more philosophical lens, these sorts of traumas might best be described as events that split life into two. Before the event, there is wholeness. After the event, there is fracture. Where there was once some semblance of safety and security, dignity and peace, there is now fear and hopelessness, pain and grief.

Even if you don't think you've experienced trauma, I'm willing to bet that, over the course of your life, you've faced major conflicts and stressors, or you've said or done things you're not proud of. Much of life is painful; we all feel guilt and shame, fear and regret. We are all searching for wholeness. And let us not forget what Victor Frankl taught us. Suffering is like a gas. There is absolutely no point to comparing traumas or shaming yourself into thinking you didn't have it bad enough for anyone to care.

— — —

I cannot and will not pretend this book offers a cure for anyone who has suffered after surviving a traumatic event. It doesn't. As Herman wisely notes, "Resolution of the trauma is never final; recovery is never complete."[10] What this book can offer is guidance, support, assistance, and care. It can help you tell your story—if that's what you want to do. I feel I must warn you, though: what we are about to begin together is not easy; it is not meant for everyone. One of my favorite authors makes this point much better than I can. "Writing isn't hard work," Philip Roth explained to an interviewer once, "it's a nightmare." As one of the most influential and prolific writers of the twentieth century, Roth knew what he was talking about. "Coal mining is hard work," he continued. "In most professions there's a beginning, a middle, and an end. With writing, it's always beginning again."[11]

If writing personal stories were easy, books like this wouldn't need to exist. It's the torturous nature of writing that has led some to conclude writing is a skill that simply cannot be taught. Another one of my all-time favorite writers, John Steinbeck, puts it this way: "If there is a magic in story writing, and I am convinced there is, no one has ever been able to reduce it to a recipe that can be passed from one person to another. The formula seems to lie solely in the aching urge of the writer to convey something he feels important to the reader."[12]

While I agree with the former point Steinbeck makes above, I must disagree with the latter. There is a science—a formula—to telling stories of trauma and transformation. In the pages that follow, I tell stories about me and my work that will take you, step by step, from the first glimmer of an idea, to an evolving, multilayered writing blueprint. My goal is to help steer you along a path that leads to a riveting and impactful story that will help change how your readers see the world. By way of detailing my own tragedies and triumphs, I attempt to define for you the barriers and challenges you will likely encounter along the way. And I try to help you overcome them, too. Near the end of this book, in a section called "Storytelling Exercises," I have included several exercises I use in my teaching that can help you turn your ideas into stories you'll be proud to share with the world.

In addition to the technical difficulties inherent in writing one's personal story, there is a chance that what you read in this book will dredge up old memories and feelings you may not know how to process. You need to be prepared for how you might react and what you will do if your feelings become overwhelming. To quote an expert in the field of expressive writing, James W. Pennebaker, "If you feel you need to write, then write. But if you feel you aren't ready, don't. If you start writing and feel you aren't making progress or you are getting more distressed, stop. Write about less emotional topics. Write about superficial issues. Don't drag yourself through the mud. You are already in the mud."[13]

It's not easy to fumble desperately along life's path, searching for some way to feel whole again. That is why I also feel compelled to say that you and you alone can decide when you are ready to transform your trauma into a meaningful story. It's not for me or anyone else to decide that for you. And it will be you and you alone who will know when you're ready to share what you've uncovered.

If while reading this book or writing about your trauma you feel as though you are in particularly bad shape—feelings of deep depression, self-destructive thoughts, potentially dangerous behaviors—please find a professional you can talk to.

About a month after my class's edited collection was published; after my student started talking to a counselor at the local VA (Veterans Affairs) hospital; after he read his revised story to a crowd of 200 friends and family members at the book's release party; after he made peace with what he had written and was acknowledged, appreciated, and understood—he came to my house one night after suppertime and knocked on my back door while I was doing dishes at the sink. I opened the door with my elbow while drying my hands. His face lit up from the kitchen light spilling through the open door. I invited him in, but he declined with a smile. "Still have that housing?" he asked. "I think I'd like it back now."

References

1. Judith Lewis Herman, *Trauma and Recovery: The Aftermath of Violence—from Domestic Abuse to Political Terror* (New York: Basic Books, 1992), 1.

2. James W. Pennebaker and Joshua M. Smyth, *Opening Up by Writing It Down: How Expressive Writing Improves Health and Eases Emotional Pain*, 3rd ed. (New York: Guilford Press, 2016), ix.

3. Viktor Frankl, *Man's Search for Meaning* (New York: Washington Square Press, 1997), 64.

4. David Chrisinger, ed., *See Me for Who I Am: Student Veterans' Stories of War and Coming Home* (Albany, NY: Hudson Whitman Press, 2016).

5. Frankl, *Man's Search for Meaning*, 100.

6. Frankl, *Man's Search for Meaning*, 101.

7. Dean G. Kilpatrick et al., "National Estimates of Exposure to Traumatic Events and PTSD Prevalence Using DSM-IV and DSM-5 Criteria," *Journal of Traumatic Stress* 26, no. 5 (2013): 537–47, https://www.ncbi.nlm.nih.gov/pmc/articles/PMC4096796/.

8. Stania Kamara et al., "Mental Health Care during the Ebola Virus Disease Outbreak in Sierra Leone," *Bulletin of the World Health Organization* 95, no. 12 (2017): 842–47, https://www.who.int/bulletin/volumes/95/12/16-190470.pdf.

9. Herman, *Trauma and Recovery*, 33.

10. Herman, *Trauma and Recovery*, 211.

11. Philip Roth quoted in *Daily Rituals: How Artists Work*, ed. Mason Currey (New York: Knopf, 2013).

12. "John Steinbeck and Advice for Beginning Writers," 1963 open letter to writers, reposted on a website, http://www.rjgeib.com/thoughts/steinbeck/steinbeck.html.

13. Pennebaker and Smyth, *Opening Up by Writing It Down*, 160.

PART I The Searching

1

Finding Your Story of Transformation

THE BLOOD pumped in my ears as a single thought raced through my mind. *They must have made a mistake letting me in.*

On the Saturday night before my first quarter of graduate classes began, three days before that first attack struck, my master's program held a student mixer in a small lounge area on the third floor of an old stone building on the southeast side of campus. I sipped fancy-tasting wine from a clear plastic cup and stood next to an assortment of food trays set on a folding table near the door. I was trying to eat as much of the free food as I could without looking like some starving vagrant who had wandered into the party by mistake.

"What are you here to study?" a new classmate of mine with a deep red tie asked me after we accidentally made eye contact while scanning the food table. "Nazi Germany," I replied. "You?" As he explained his planned research project, I nodded politely but wasn't able to follow along with much of what he said. Then he asked me what specifically I was going to study about Nazi Germany, and I told him I was interested in telling the stories of people who survived the Nazi years in hiding, those who would have been persecuted and most likely murdered for who they were. Many of the survivors I had read about before coming to the University of Chicago felt a deep sense of shame at having survived when so many others had not. He suggested I take a look at the diary of a Jewish man who had hidden in France during the Nazi years, and I told him that sounded perfect but that I couldn't read French. He looked surprised. "How are you going to study European history if you can't read one of the major European languages?" he asked.

On the morning the attack struck, I felt like I'd just stepped off a spinning ride at a carnival even though I was simply sitting at the kitchen table checking my email. When the weight of everything that lay ahead of me morphed into a literal weight that started to crush my chest, I began to sob, my tears plunking onto the keys of my laptop. My wife, Ashley, heard me and darted out of our bedroom. We'd been together for four years and married only a couple of months, and she had seen me cry on only one other occasion. She didn't hesitate. She didn't even ask me what was wrong. Before I could squeeze out a few words to tell her I was fine, she bear-hugged me from behind. Her chest smashed up against my shoulder blades; her chin dug into the space between my neck and shoulder. "Match my breathing," she said, as she pulled my body even closer to her own. "Breathe like I breathe."

— — —

By the time my wife and I received the wedding invitation from Whitney and Brett, I was feeling much more confident that I'd somehow survive graduate school. Their invitation surprised me for a couple of reasons. First, it said that Brett would be deploying to Afghanistan a week and a half after the wedding, and second, Brett and I had seen each other only a handful of times—usually when he was home on leave between deployments—since he'd left for boot camp a couple of weeks before I left for college. Each time we ran into each other, it felt to me as though we'd drifted farther and farther apart.

Brett wore his dress blues for the ceremony, and the low-hanging autumn sun lit up his bride-to-be in her white dress. During the reception, in between the "Chicken Dance" and "Cotton Eye Joe," I found Brett leaning against a post in the corner of the reception tent. He asked me about graduate school as he scanned the dancing crowd. I didn't tell him about my panic attacks.

"I'm surviving," I said, immediately regretting my poor choice of words.

He locked eyes with me for a moment when I asked about Afghanistan. Then he looked down at the Solo cup of beer he'd been sipping; it seemed like he was sick of people asking him about his upcoming deployment. After a moment, he told me he'd gotten hooked up with a great gig. Probably wouldn't see much action, he said. I smiled and nodded, unsure how to respond without making more of an ass of myself.

Back in Chicago, I got into the habit of watching the WGN channel while Ashley made dinner most nights. Sometimes there'd be a short segment about a Marine or two who'd been killed by an IED in southern Afghanistan, and I would wonder about Brett. I hated myself for thinking that what I was going through at school was so difficult compared to what he was enduring.

When we were both still in high school, Brett and I had talked about enlisting together, but my father talked me out of it. While I was in my freshman year of college, I had planned instead to enroll in ROTC (Reserve Officers' Training Corps), but Ashley, who had decided in the first month of dating me that we would be getting married someday, talked me out of that. Sitting on the couch in my apartment, trying to imagine what Brett was going through, I felt the shame of not having enlisted with him that usually turned into an anxious fear: if Brett made it home alive, and if I finished graduate school, he and I would no longer have anything in common—nothing to keep us connected.

How Do You Know If You Have a Story to Tell?

The main difference between a story and an anecdote is that a story shows transformation over time. And the only thing that causes transformation is conflict. Think for a moment about something from your past that you might want to write about. Was there something you wanted that you had to struggle to get? Were there any obstacles, challenges, or antagonists that tried to stop you from getting what you wanted? Was there a moment when all seemed lost, when it seemed like quitting was the only option? Were you able to overcome those forces opposed to you? If you answered yes to these questions, you absolutely have a story to tell that is more complicated than simply what happened to you. Your story is a detailed retelling of how the things that happened to you affected you, what hard decision you made in the face of conflict and struggle, and how you changed or what you learned as a result.

I know what you might be thinking. What if you can't find the right words? What if you have so many words that you don't know where to begin? The process we are about to begin can help you with both problems by helping you narrow down the number of stories that you could tell until you arrive at *your* story. How will you know when you find it? That's the easy part: It will feel the most honest. It will settle into your heart. It will feel like the truth. It will allow you to feel whole, to start a new beginning.

— — —

About 15 months after Brett and Whitney's wedding, Ashley and I were living in Washington, DC, expecting our first child. I had finished my master's program the year Brett was in Afghanistan, and he and I hadn't seen each other since he'd left for his deployment. Sitting on the floor of my bedroom just after midnight one cold night in February, unable to sleep, I flipped open my laptop and logged on to Facebook. Brett was logged on too, so I sent him a message and asked how he was doing. He began typing. "Not that good, man," he wrote. "I think I'm kinda fucked up."

A wave of panic started in my stomach and bubbled up into my chest. *Don't write anything stupid,* I thought. Seconds passed. It felt like forever. Brett's typing bubble popped up again. I took a deep breath. He was really struggling, he wrote. He had frequent panic attacks. He couldn't shake whatever was going on. He was drinking too much and missed being with his guys. Whitney just didn't get it, he said.

When I called him the next day to continue our conversation, he was surprised to hear from me. He hadn't remembered our middle-of-the-night chat. "I was pretty drunk last night," he confessed. What he told me next was that he hadn't been anything but tired and numb for the past year or so and that he had lost a lot, seen far too much, but was missing it all badly. He couldn't shake the images of the body splayed out on the floor of the armored troop carrier, known in the military as an MRAP, and he tempered any resulting depression by trying to remind himself how lucky he was never to have had to put a best friend in a body bag—or be put in one himself. Yet the guilt of surviving sometimes remained.

"I feel like part of me died over there," he told me a few days later. "The old me is either dead or fucked up at least," he explained, "but I would do it all again in a heartbeat. I guess that's the fucked-up thing about war. You'd do it all again, even knowing everything you know after."

For the next couple of weeks, Brett and I talked on the phone almost daily. I was worried about him. Talking seemed to help him, but it was hard to make the time, and there were topics I felt too nervous to ask him about. We started emailing regularly instead. Brett told me about the battle for Marjah, and I had to admit I'd never heard of Marjah. I could tell my ignorance was hard for him to understand. Not wanting to make him ever feel like that again, I headed to the library down the road from my apartment whenever I had a spare hour or two. If I had a question about something I was reading, I'd send an email to Brett and ask him about it. He became my subject matter expert. I became his sounding board.

— — —

Halfway through June the year that Brett and I reconnected on Facebook, I flew back home to Wisconsin and told Brett I'd stop in to see him while I was around. The night we met for beers at a restaurant near his home, he wore a dark T-shirt, jeans, and a white baseball cap with a curved brim, which he'd pulled down low over his eyes. His hair was cropped close to his head, a stark contrast to the scraggly black beard that covered his rough and angular chin. His eyes were puffy and tired, and even after he settled into his seat at the table, his shoulders stayed pulled up, almost to his ears.

Just like that night on Facebook, we didn't waste time with small talk. Brett tried not to think too much about Afghanistan, he said, but most of the time he couldn't help it. Memories of his convoy being ambushed and the distressed cries that rose from the mound of mangled bodies in the back of the MRAP would play in his mind against his will. While he talked, he mostly looked at the tall can of Miller Lite he was almost strangling with his calloused hands. Occasionally he'd whip his head around to check what was going on behind him.

He told me that no one wanted to hear the truth about what he had been through, that he usually broke into a panic he tried desperately to conceal whenever anyone asked too many questions. Everyone in his life seemed to have made up their minds about the war, he thought. And if it came up at all, Brett could tell that what they really wanted was some confirmation of what they already believed. If they thought the war was a waste, Brett would tell them stories about the mind-numbing boredom or about the money that was being wasted or about how unprepared the Afghan National Army was to take over the fight against the Taliban. If they thought the opposite, Brett could tell them stories about the incremental progress being made and about how Marjah, a Taliban stronghold, had fallen and how the Marines were never going to give it up.

In the middle of detailing the worst days of his life to me, Brett would occasionally look up from his beer to see how I was reacting. I made a point not to look away. Even though our lives had diverged after high school, Brett was still my friend. I needed him to know that, but I struggled to find the right words. Instead, whenever he looked at me, I locked eyes with him, surrendering to the indescribable telepathy that had taken hold of us. I needed him to know that there was nothing he could say to make me think less of him.

"Sharing the traumatic experience with others," writes Judith Herman, "is a precondition for the restitution of a sense of a meaningful world. In this process, the survivor seeks assistance not only from those closest to her but also from the wider community. The response of the community depends, first, upon public acknowledgment of the traumatic event and, second, upon some form of community action."[1]

I didn't bear-hug Brett that night at the restaurant or ask him to breathe like I was breathing, but in my own way, by listening to him, without trying to fix anything, I hoped he felt as much relief as I had when Ashley had reminded me back in graduate school that I too wasn't alone.

— — —

January 9th used to be an ordinary date on the calendar. That all changed for Brett in 2010. Ever since then, that infamous date sticks up from the calendar like a rusty nail, a marker for a memory of the day that a 23-year-old Marine and an embedded journalist were killed and six other Marines were seriously wounded. It happened on a gravel road near Nawa, in southern Afghanistan, where insurgents buried 500 pounds of explosives that tossed the 18-ton MRAP 35 feet in the air.

"It was a hot day, and I was riding in a convoy of seven MRAP trucks," Brett told me. MRAP stands for "mine-resistant ambush pro-tected," and these heavily armored vehicles are designed specifically to withstand the blast of an IED. "We were on our way to a patrol base in Helmand province. My team leader and I were in Vic 2," meaning the second vehicle in the convoy.

"That day started out innocently enough," he continued. "We began our trip just like we had dozens of times before. I remember noticing the farmland and irrigation canals and the little clay huts the Afghans lived in as we slowly crawled along the countryside."

Then came the explosion.

"For a moment, I looked around, a little unsure about what had hap-pened exactly. Suddenly, a voice came over the radio: 'Vic 6 got hit! Vic 6 got hit!'"

"At first, I couldn't really believe what was happening," Brett con-tinued. "The IED had enough force that it actually picked up the vehi-cle and tossed it into a ditch, where we found it lying on its side. The vehicle's back axle had been blown off and debris littered the ground around it. The first casualty I noticed was the truck's gunner. He was lying on the ground, unconscious but alive."

After arriving at the damaged vehicle, Brett and his team leader found the driver and the front-seat passenger alive and moaning in pain. "My team leader and our radio operator tried to pull the driver out while I ran to the back of the truck to open the two main doors to the passenger area," Brett remembered. "But since the axle was blown off, and because the truck was dug into the ground, I couldn't pry the doors open more than a couple of inches. With the door cracked open, though, I could hear the moaning of those trapped inside."

Once Brett gave up on trying to pry the back doors open, he saw that the driver of the truck had been pulled from his seat, so he ran around to that side of the truck and jumped inside. "I made my way to the back passenger area," he said. "The seats were ripped off the brackets and thrown across the compartment, and there were bodies lying everywhere." He paused for a moment. A vacant stare came across his face. "Just this heap of stuff," he continued. "The first Marine I pulled out was young. Blood pooled from his mouth, and he had a big gash on his leg. He tried to say something—it sounded like 'Help me,' but I can't be sure."

Brett made several trips back into the truck to pull out wounded Marines. One had two broken ankles. Another was likely suffering from internal hemorrhaging. Then he saw that the British photographer who had been riding along with them that day was seriously injured. "His legs were crushed by a pile of debris," Brett remembered. He sipped from his beer and took a deep breath. "I knew I wouldn't be able to pull him out myself, so I yelled for someone to help me. Then I realized his legs were twisted backward and caught under a seat."

As Brett and another Marine dragged the photographer out of the truck by his vest, Brett noticed that the pile of debris he had been climbing over on each of his trips in and out of the MRAP was concealing a body. "I knew there was a dead body under there," he told me, "but I stopped for a moment and checked for a pulse anyway." Another long pause. "Nothing." The body Brett discovered belonged to Rupert Hamer, a seasoned combat journalist from London and the first British journalist to be killed in Afghanistan.

"Once we had everybody out of the truck," Brett said, "I crawled out and saw bodies scattered all over the road. After looking around for a few seconds, I noticed the Marine who had the nasty gash on his leg. Our radio operator had placed a tourniquet around his leg, but that gash was the least of his injuries. He wasn't breathing."

Once a medevac helicopter arrived, the Marines on the ground loaded the wounded onto stretchers. "It was then that I noticed a few Marines had pulled out the dead body I had found inside the truck," Brett continued. "I ran over to lend a hand. I stood to the side of the truck as the other Marines lowered the body down from the roof. We laid him on a stretcher and placed a blanket over him."

"Before we finished," he continued, "I noticed one of the corpsmen had broken down. He was crying. It wasn't a sad cry, though—there was more rage than sadness. I didn't know what to do, so I just knelt down for a moment. I started shaking and couldn't stop." Brett paused, took the last sip from his beer and motioned to the waitress to bring another. "The adrenaline of the situation was starting to wear off," he said. "It wasn't until that moment that I noticed my hands, my pants, and my flak jacket—everything—was covered with blood."

— — —

More than 7,000 miles away from Afghanistan in Wisconsin, Brett's wife was hoping that day would be a day she would get to talk to Brett. "Communication was minimal," she told me about their time apart. "I remember clinging to my cell phone everywhere I went, sitting by the computer hoping to catch him on chat, staying up until four a.m. because of the time difference, checking my email 24-7." Whitney's life had become a tunnel with Brett at the end of it. To act carefree like everyone else took nearly all the strength she had. Alone. Empty. Her body was at home, at work, or at school, but her mind and heart, as well as her soul, were with Brett. "It was beyond difficult," Whitney continued, "to carry on with my schoolwork, my work, family, and friends and not let it show that I was upset or worried or scared. I was pretty much in my own world for the entire time he was deployed and an entirely different person when he was home safe."

When Brett was in Iraq in 2007, he would sometimes go a month or longer without communicating with Whitney. And when they did talk, Brett kept most of the bad stuff to himself; he didn't want to make her worry. Before he left for Afghanistan, though, Whitney made it clear to him that holding stuff back wasn't going to fly this time around and that she did not want him to withhold anything.

The night after his convoy was ambushed, Brett carved out some time to call Whitney on the satellite phone. "I could hear it in his voice more than ever that something terrible had happened," Whitney told me, tears welling up in her blue-gray eyes, "and he told me a little but not nearly as much as I learned once he returned home. He just told me that there was an explosion and that a bunch of guys didn't make it, that it was bad . . . really bad. My heart was breaking for him. It was very difficult to hear his voice, know that he was hurting, and not be able to do anything about it."

When Brett left for Afghanistan, Whitney worried that he might not come home at all. Brett worried about that, too, at least at first. After that fateful day in January 2010, Whitney began to worry about how Brett would be changed by all he was forced to endure. "I knew that I would never fully understand what had happened, never feel his pain," Whitney confided in me. "I was so thankful he was okay, but I knew at the same time that someone else had just lost someone they loved and that Brett would be changed forever."

— — —

All the research I did in the months after Brett and I had started talking again taught me one thing above all else: Brett's story was far from unique. Thousands of America's post-9/11 veterans have recurrent and intrusive memories of their trauma, even years later, which many will do almost anything to avoid. They find it hard to sleep or turn off the hypervigilance they relied on to stay alive overseas. Many are paranoid and quick to anger. Countless more come back with post-traumatic stress, a term used to describe those who, like Brett, tested below a diagnostic threshold but who have symptoms of post-traumatic stress disorder that are strong enough to disrupt their daily lives. Above all else, Brett felt unsafe and alienated, even among those who loved him most. "I was always sizing people up," Brett told me, "assessing threats, planning escapes. I would think constantly about how I would disable an attacker. What if someone was waiting for me around the corner? Outside my home? I felt like I had to be ready all the time."

Despite the undeniable hellishness of what he experienced in Afghanistan, perhaps what was most difficult for Brett was replacing the sense of purpose he felt while deployed. For many veterans, it's not necessarily the trauma of war that affects them most, but rather they miss what's *good* about being at war—for lack of a better term—once they return home. What few civilians realize is that for most veterans, their military service was not simply a job—it was an identity. With each deployment, each combat experience, each trauma endured, that identity becomes more and more entrenched. "When I left the Marine Corps, I felt lost, confused, and angry," Brett told me a couple of years after he got out. That feeling of loss, confusion, and anger wasn't easy to deal with, either. Brett thought drinking would help. Soon enough, by his own estimation, he became a "sleep-deprived, anxious, alcoholic mess who couldn't maintain a decent relationship with his wife."

After feeling like he was going somewhere for five years while in the Marine Corps, Brett suddenly found himself on the outside, seemingly going nowhere. While enclosed in the Corps' universe of regimented life—shit, shower, shave, train for war, go to war, survive, memorialize, return—Brett had a meaningful place in an institution that was greater than he was. The second he took off his uniform for the last time, however, he felt like less than nothing. "My status vanished instantly," he told me. "I had no direction, no purpose."

— — —

Some years ago, I read a book titled *The Heart and the Fist*, which was written by a humanitarian with a doctorate from Oxford University who later became a Navy SEAL after he became convinced that humanitarianism couldn't exist without military force. At one point in the book, the author details a trip he took to Bethesda Naval Hospital to visit wounded Marines after he had returned from a deployment to Iraq. What struck him most about the men he met that day was their unwavering desire to continue serving their country, despite all they had already given—and lost. Seeing such determination reminded the author of the time he had spent working with refugees before he joined the Navy. "To build a new life in the face of great challenge," he wrote, "what mattered was not what we gave them but what they did."[2] It wasn't long before the author had an idea that became a part-time project and eventually grew into The Mission Continues, a national nonprofit service organization that helps veterans transition from the military to service and leadership programs where they can continue to serve in their communities. "Veterans possess the drive and desire to serve others," he writes, "but without access to the tools needed, their potential to make meaningful impact at the local level remains untapped."[3]

The author, who went on to become the governor of Missouri, has fallen from grace since his book came out, but that shouldn't discount what he saw and wrote about, nor should it take anything away from the impact his book had on me all those years ago. When I told Brett about all the amazing work The Mission Continues was doing with transitioning veterans, something clicked inside his head.

"Let's try to raise some money for them," he suggested to me on the phone a few days before Christmas in 2012. "What if we run a marathon or something?"

I thought for a moment.

"What if," I said, "we ran a 50-mile ultramarathon instead?"

What's Your Story of Transformation?

That a survivor of trauma could *grow* as a result of the experience was put on an academic footing by Richard Tedeschi, a professor emeritus of psychology at the University of North Carolina at Charlotte. In the early 1990s, Tedeschi interviewed people who had sustained severe physical injuries, including several people who had been paralyzed in car accidents. He also interviewed senior citizens who had outlived their longtime spouses. What Tedeschi found was that the people he interviewed believed that even though they regretted the loss of their mobility or their spouse, their traumatic experience had led to positive transformation and had given them a fresh perspective on life.[4]

When I teach storytelling to military veterans and their families, my first goal is to help them think more clearly—and zero in quickly—on ways they may have changed or grown because of a traumatic or harrowing experience by having them fill out what I call a Transformation Inventory. The inventory (modified from Tedeschi's research findings) lists 18 common ways that people have reported changing as a result of surviving trauma. These ways can be grouped into the following areas:

- *New Possibilities*: "I can now do better things with my life."
- *Increased Strength*: "I am stronger than I thought I was."
- *More Meaningful Relationships*: "I can count on people in times of trouble."
- *Greater Appreciation*: "I better appreciate the value of my own life."
- *Spiritual Development*: "I have a stronger religious or spiritual faith."

I ask my seminar participants to read the inventory and think about ways they might have changed because of a traumatic or difficult situation. If they experienced one change to a great degree, I ask them to take note of that because there is, without a doubt, the makings of a story that needs to be told.

You can try taking the inventory yourself (first in the section "Storytelling Exercises"). Not everyone will experience change in every area, of course. In fact, I've never worked with a writer who reported experiencing a great degree of change in every area of the Transformation Inventory. What is likely to happen is that you'll note transformation in two or three areas that generally relate to one another. You may find, for example, that your traumatic experience led to new possibilities for your life and made you realize you were stronger than you thought you were. Or your experiences led you to form more meaningful relationships and helped you find greater appreciation of your life.

Once you've finished filling out the Transformation Inventory, pick one to three of the areas you marked as ones of significant change and add them to the end of the following phrase: "I believe . . ." You might write, for example, "I believe I am stronger than I thought I was and have more compassion for others." Knowing what you believe is important because once you know that, you can then begin answering two questions that will help you *show* what you believe to a reader.

The first question you need to answer is "How so?" How did you come to believe you can now do better things with your life? How are you stronger than you thought you were? How did you come to realize you can count on others in a time of trouble? How did you come to have a better appreciation of the value of your life? How has your faith been strengthened?

It's at this point in the writing process where you can begin forming a timeline. At the right end of that timeline is your eventual transformation as a result of the trauma you endured. If you can determine what should go at the left end of that timeline—the beginning—you will have a better sense of who you were before you experienced your trauma. The second, and admittedly much more difficult, question to answer is "Why?" Why did you change as a result of your experience? Why did you decide to do something different, to be someone different?

— — —

Once Brett and I got to the 36-mile mark of the 50-mile ultramarathon, we both had entered uncharted territory. Neither one of us had ever run so far. And neither one of us knew how our bodies were going to respond. With every stride, we were redefining what was possible.

"I think I'm burning my matches," I told Brett between heavy breaths.

There's an adage in endurance racing that says all runners start a race with a metaphorical book of matches. Whenever runners put forth an effort that exceeds what they can sustain evenly from start to finish, they burn a match. There are only so many matches to burn, and when they're gone, they're gone.

"Grin and bear it," Brett told me. "Just grin and bear it."

After more than eight hours of running, there was a fierce battle being waged in each of our minds. In one trench was the suffering, the pain. And in the other, an intense desire to resist the impulse to quit. Brett was suppressing the pain he felt in his ankle and hips. I was fighting to ignore the cramping in my hamstrings. We both fought to keep food down and to stay hydrated. Running an ultramarathon—like combat in so many ways—is a "fight or flight" situation, plain and simple. Our sympathetic nervous systems were shunting blood away from our stomachs and intestines and toward the muscles in our legs, as well as to our lungs, hearts, and brains. At the same time, the pounding of our feet on the cold pavement was raising the pressure in our stomach cavities to two or three times the normal level. By the time we got to the 28-mile mark, I couldn't keep any solid food down; I tried drinking chicken broth, but even that came right back up.

With about 10 miles to go, I did the math and realized that unless Brett and I picked up the pace, we weren't going to finish before the 11-hour cutoff. The race's website said that after 11 hours, all finishers would still get a finisher's medal but would not get an "official time." As far as the race director was concerned, if we couldn't finish in less than 11 hours, we shouldn't have been out there in the first place. While I was calculating split times, Brett was falling into the darkness of his own mind. Overcome with negative thoughts, he was burning matches. All he wanted was to stop.

With five miles to go, we reached the last checkpoint. Whitney was there to greet us. She could see how drained Brett was feeling. And like that morning in my apartment, when Ashley helped me through my first panic attack, Whitney hugged Brett tightly and whispered into his ear something that seemed to dissipate whatever gloomy feelings Brett was struggling with. He suddenly looked lighter and powerful. "What did you say?" I asked her, as Brett headed back toward the road. Whitney turned to me with a smile: "Remember what you're doing this for!"

That was when everything clicked inside his head, Brett told me after the race: "All the darkness went away, and I thought, 'She's right; there are guys that would kill to be able to use their legs again or take another step, or hug their children, or hold their wives. Some of them will never be able to do that again, so what the fuck do I have to complain about? Yeah, your legs are hurting a bit; get over it and suck it the fuck up.'" With only a few miles to go, Brett thought about all the men he had deployed with and all the good times they'd had together. He thought about all the people in his life who loved him and supported him. He was determined not to let any of them down.

"I'll be fine," I shouted to him when he stopped and looked back at me from the road. "You go—I'll be right behind you." It was a lie. I knew I wouldn't be able to keep up with him. My legs were drained of life, and every time I tried to dig deep, the meat in my hamstrings turned to stone.

"The pain just went away," Brett told me a few days after the race, "My legs, my hips, my ankle, all the pain just stopped. So I took off. I ran from mile marker to mile marker. I couldn't believe what was happening and how good I felt. I thought, 'Holy shit, I'm really gonna make it.'" Through sheer force of will, Brett tapped into something he didn't even know he had. He covered the last five miles in 40 minutes, an amazing show of mental and physical toughness for anyone—let alone someone who had already been running for over 10 hours.

As he approached the finish line, Brett was overcome with a sense of calm. "I remember thinking that this was awesome," he said, "and that I didn't remember too many times in my life when I'd felt like that. I was proud of myself for doing it and honored that I got to share the experience with such great people." The person Brett had become at that moment was the best possible version of himself, the person he wanted to be all his life. No regrets. No hesitations. His old life—with all its hurt and pain—fell away. It was gone, at least for a little while. He felt free. That's what running an ultramarathon does, we discovered. Each race offers its own experience, its own story, and its own lasting life change.

Then there was me. As day gave way to dusk, my race began its descent. I was trying to come to terms with the fact that I was going to have to cover the last five miles on my own. Pulling out of the last aid station, my legs wouldn't move beyond a slow grind. Unable to eat or drink, I braced myself for that voice of doubt and negativity that shows up whenever life gets overwhelming, the voice that tells me I don't belong, that I'm not good enough.

My legs felt heavier with each plodding step. I felt light-headed, and my vision was blurry, like a punch-drunk boxer seconds before the final blow. I was looking at my feet as they seemed to sink into the pavement, wondering which step would be my last, when my wife ran up from behind and slapped me on the ass.

"All we have left is 4.7. We can do it!"

With that slap, I suddenly felt lighter, as though I had thrown off a weighted vest. My wife, who was four months pregnant with our second child at the time, wasn't about to let me go it alone. My feet switched back and forth, almost effortlessly.

"Tough as nails," she said. "You're tough as nails."

In a 50-mile ultramarathon, runners compete against their own limits, not against anyone else. To finish is to win. Such is true in life as well. With about three miles to go, a Zen-like feeling washed over me. All the clutter and noise and frustration and responsibility of my life were suddenly gone. There was no yesterday. There was no tomorrow. There was only that moment, that joy.

At six feet four inches and 240 pounds, I've gotten incredulous looks at nearly every endurance race I've ever run. The day we ran that ultramarathon, however, Brett and I did something that not many people can say they have done. We started running at seven o'clock, and we didn't stop until we crossed the finish line 50 miles down the road. One thing I desperately wanted was to finish in less than 11 hours. I crossed the line in 11 hours and 14 minutes. No official finish time for me. Even so, I wasn't upset. Far from it. When I crossed the finish line, Brett was there to greet me. We hugged each other, and all the emotions of the day came flooding over us. I didn't want to let go. I wanted to remember every feeling, every sensation. We had suffered together. We had hurt together. And in that moment we were triumphant together.

The experience taught me two things. The first is that suffering is humbling—and sometimes it can even be necessary. The second is that in running ultramarathons, you don't have to be fast. All you must be is fearless. You must be fearless because you can't know how hard it's going to be. Endurance running is a lot like writing—and life—for that matter. All you can do is show up, toe the start line, control what you can control, and not worry about the rest.

References

1. Judith Lewis Herman, *Trauma and Recovery: The Aftermath of Violence—from Domestic Abuse to Political Terror* (New York: Basic Books, 1992), 70.

2. Eric Greitens, *The Heart and the Fist: The Education of a Humanitarian, the Making of a Navy SEAL* (New York: Houghton Mifflin Harcourt, 2011), 290.

3. "About Us," The Mission Continues, https://missioncontinues.org/about/.

4. Posttraumatic Growth Research Group, Department of Psychological Science, University of North Carolina at Charlotte, https://ptgi.uncc.edu/.

2

Uncovering Your Object of Desire

I WANTED TO pinch Robert's tiny crimson foot. I wanted to hear him cry. After all the uncertainty and dashed hopes, after all the fear and suffering, Robert Louis Chrisinger came into the world without a sound. Without the joy of being alive. After all this time, it's that silent sadness that sticks with me most of all. I didn't expect stillness. I expected the maniacal beeping of vital monitors and the dull hum of overhead lamps. On that humid summer night in 2017, the night we lost Robert, the nurses didn't need the monitors. The doctor didn't need the lamps. There was no need to search for signals of something going wrong. There was no need to analyze and reassure.

I sat scrunched on a chair next to the hospital bed, leaning over with my elbows on my knees, holding my wife's hand in mine as the doctor conducted her examination. "I'm so, so sorry," the doctor said behind her surgical mask. "I'm so sorry this is happening to you."

Because she was only halfway through her pregnancy, Ashley would probably need to push only once or twice, the doctor said. Ashley nodded; I squeezed her hand. As the next contraction began, Ashley curled up into a fist, pushing her heels into the foot of the bed. Once the vise released her, Robert slipped out, and the rock-hard pain of contraction lifted as suddenly as it had arrived. In her floating sense of physical relief, Ashley wept.

—— —— ——

Half a year passed before I worked up the nerve to look through the photos the nurse had taken of Robert on the day he was born. When she asked Ashley and me if we wanted her to take the pictures, we politely declined her offer. Neither one of us could believe that anyone would want photographic evidence of such a devastating loss.

But after all we had endured—rushing to the emergency room in the middle of the night, conversing with several specialists who couldn't explain why this was happening to us, wringing our hands for a week in a hospital room reserved for mothers who were losing their babies, and finding a glimmer of hope when the early labor had stalled—we relented. There was no more fight in us. We were as limp as pie dough, slumped against each other as the nurse powered on her digital camera. "I know it doesn't feel like it now," she said, "but everything happens for a reason. This is all part of God's plan."

Robert's skin was pink at first. His tiny eyes were fused shut; his ears were pinned to his head. As the nurse clicked away, Robert's skin turned crimson, becoming stickier and translucent. When I held him, the blanket the doctor had wrapped him in felt rough from too many washings. I fought the urge to imagine how raw he would have felt if he were still alive. The medical literature I read months after we lost Robert said babies as young as he was cannot feel pain. I hope that's true.

After I handed Robert back to Ashley, she laid him in her lap and studied him with weary eyes. She seemed transfixed, awestruck by his tiny fingers, his clear toenails, and the grace of his bony shoulders. She then picked him up and held him close to her chest, as if all he needed was some motherly love. The shutter clicked again as I tried for the last time to think of something encouraging to say, something wise and useful enough to untangle the dark knot I could sense forming in the pit of Ashley's stomach.

The entire time Ashley had been pregnant with Robert, her pregnancy had felt provisional and precarious. Every cramp or twinge of pain she felt ushered in uncertainty and fear. Because we had already lost two pregnancies to miscarriage, the scales seemed tipped toward further heartbreak. We were careful not to tell anyone we were trying again. Certainty was a vapor. We didn't say a word about Robert until Ashley was about 15 weeks along, after our doctor had told us everything was looking fine. She said we had nothing to worry about.

The shutter clicked one last time as I told Ashley I thought she was wonderful and brave. Stronger than I've ever been. Despite all that had happened, I still felt a twinge of pride when I looked at her. A bleak pride. A heart-twisting pride that ached inside my chest. In the resulting picture, Ashley is marooned on the bed, staring at me with a stunned look, confusion mixed with incredulity bordering on horror. In that moment, I felt so ineffectual, so out of place. What love and encouragement I could muster in that moment simply wasn't enough to stop her cascade of suffering.

Logically, I knew that Robert was not a fully formed human being, that he was merely the possibility of a person. At the same time, I felt gutted thinking about having to rise to my feet and walk together with Ashley into a world that Robert would never know.

— — —

I had not written a word about Robert until the last full day of a week-long writing seminar I taught in November 2018. Nor had I planned to write about him, either. I thought at the time that my despair was still too mountainous. But then one of the participants in the seminar confided in me the details of a story she desperately wanted to make sense of—and everything changed.

Sara is tall, like me, and slender, like I was before college football left me with a bad back and 50 extra pounds. Her hair is brown and shoulder length, her eyes blue and piercing. She has pronounced cheekbones and pale skin, and when she smiles, her right eyebrow arches higher than her left. Even though, like me, she is prone to melancholy and can be laceratingly self-critical, she is one of the kindest people I've ever known and has a magical skill for making others feel comfortable in even the most distressing situations.

The story Sara wanted to write at the seminar is not an easy one. When she was still in high school, she discovered she was pregnant, and because she had convinced herself that she was "unfit" to be a mother at such a young age, she placed the child for adoption. After high school, she joined the Army and deployed to Iraq, where she produced video news packages about her fellow soldiers and coalition forces working together to rebuild Iraq's war-damaged infrastructure. Sara is a survivor of military sexual trauma and an open book when it comes to discussing her post-traumatic stress.

A few months after she returned from her last deployment, Sara met and fell in love with a fellow Iraq War veteran named Andy. She told herself that she had been waiting for someone like Andy, someone she could start a family with and prove, once and for all, her fitness as a mother. Once they began trying to conceive, however, Sara learned that she would likely never be able to birth another child. Fortunately, Sara and her husband were afforded the opportunity to adopt a little boy.

She told me all of this in a common area near a stone fireplace in one of the dorm buildings where she and the other seminar participants stayed during the week. She wasn't sure where to begin her story, she told me, and she wasn't sure how to end it either.

"That's simple," I said in my calm and practiced professorial tone. "What did you want? What was your fundamental goal? Was it to be a mother? To find unconditional love? To atone for whatever guilt you felt after placing your child for adoption?"

I paused, waiting for her reply. The silence felt heavy. Sara took a deep breath; her moist eyes darted to the upper corner of the room above my left shoulder. An open notebook blanketed her lap; her hands gripped its front and back covers.

"I think what I wanted was to be seen as fit," she finally said, returning her gaze to me.

"What do you mean by 'fit'?"

"Like when I was a teenager," Sara continued, "I wasn't ready to be a mother. I wasn't fit. And then, when I was in the military, the whole point of everything you do is to be 'fit for duty.' And the things that make you fit for duty are not necessarily the same characteristics or qualities that make you fit to be a mother."

"Tell me more about that," I said. The words sounded painfully hackneyed as they left my mouth. I was suddenly worried our conversation was beginning to stray into an informal therapy session.

"When Andy and I started the process of adopting, I had to meet one on one with a social worker who was there to determine whether I should be able to adopt a baby," Sara began, "and I was so worried that all of the stuff that had happened with my pregnancy and the sexual trauma I experienced in the military and all the mental health issues I had afterwards were going to affect her decision. I was scared this social worker was going to tell me I wasn't fit to be a parent, still."

She sniffled. Her cheeks tinted suddenly with glowing pink patches as the memories swam behind her eyes.

"So you wanted to be 'fit,'" I said. I felt a lump of muted anguish in my throat as I contemplated what to say next. "Start there," I finally said. "Start with the idea that you weren't fit to be a mother when you were a teenager and how you had to steel yourself against the types of thoughts and behaviors that would make you unfit as a soldier and how those experiences suddenly became possible liabilities when you started the adoption process. Without a goal like that—a goal you're trying to achieve—the story will fall flat. It won't have an arc." She was scribbling in her notebook, moving as quickly as I spoke. "The end of your story," I continued, "comes when you either get what you wanted, don't get what you wanted, or stop wanting it altogether."

When she finished writing, Sara's hands dropped into her lap like fallen logs. Conversations like these can be as physically taxing as they are emotionally.

"I lost a child, too," I said after a beat. Sara's pale lips pulled tightly against her teeth; she straightened her hunched spine. "Last summer.

My wife went into early labor; doctors don't know why." Unable to hold myself back, I told Sara that I had been trying to figure out how to write about Robert but that the narrative in my head didn't make enough sense and that I wasn't sure where to start.

"Well," she said, "what did you want?"

——— ——— ———

In the weeks that followed our loss of Robert, I found a way to resume my life in a universe that felt irrevocably different. Well-meaning friends and family tried to soften a grief I found unbearable. Some reminded me that at least Ashley and I both had our health or that we already had two beautiful children. Some told us to be thankful for what we had and told me they would pray for my strength or some other platitude. One person told me that someday I'd look back on the day we lost Robert and realize it was the start of something better.

When anyone asked me what had happened, I would rely on my own platitudes. It was bad luck, I would say. "Having bad luck" was not the answer most people I spoke to expected to hear. They were not comfortable with my conviction that Ashley and I were not in control of what happened to us. They wanted to know whether I thought the doctor was incompetent. "Did Ashley *take* anything?" one whispered to me. Others wondered, beyond earshot of Ashley, whether this tragedy could have been avoided if I hadn't let her hike 30 miles with her sister and cousin on the Appalachian Trail during the first trimester.

It seemed to me that Ashley and I were being made to believe either that we had no control and so had to submit to some higher power or that we had all the control and had failed. I eventually refused to talk to anyone about what had happened, drawing into myself like a clam inside its shell.

There were times when I wondered whether I even had the right to form memories of Robert. There were times when I felt like I was grieving the loss of something I never really had, and I couldn't make sense of that. Other times I wondered what he would have been like.

Would he have been thick bodied like me? Or would he have been long and lean like his mother? Blue eyes or brown?

What did I want? That's simple. To this day I want so badly to feel his breath on my bare chest as he naps there under a warm blanket. I want to teach him how to build a tower of blocks and to dribble a basketball. I want to read him bedtime stories and draw pictures with him at the dining room table and push him in a sled down the hill at my mother's house. I want to hear him giggle and talk in his sleep and yell out for a wipe or a Band-Aid or for help with fractions.

I want my son.

What Is Your Object of Desire?

How about you? What do you want? Whatever it is—and your pursuit to achieve it—can help establish the structure of your story. You want something, but you cannot have it right away. You must endeavor and struggle and overcome barriers that stand in your way. What will interest your readers—and hold their attention—is the conflict that arises for you as you strive for what you want.

In action stories, for example, the main character wants to succeed at something, but others want the character to fail. In a horror story, the others want something for the main character much worse than failure—damnation and death. In a crime story, the main character fights injustice in search of the truth. Thrillers are a combination of action, horror, and crime. In a classic "war" story, on the other hand, the main character struggles with wanting righteousness and becoming corrupted. In performance stories, the main character wants respect and fears being shamed, and in a love story, the main character wants, well, love.

Focusing on this struggle to get what you wanted is what will endear you to your readers. They will attach themselves to you, the narrator, because they will begin to want what you want—and they'll want to see if you get it, or not. This is why we react strongly as readers when characters in the stories we read make what seem to us to be stupid decisions. Whenever you feel yourself getting stuck, come back to your object of desire. Have you made it clear to readers what you want? Have you showed them what you did to get it?

If you turn to the end of this book, where the storytelling exercises are located, you'll find an exercise I use with writers called Your Object of Desire. In a series of steps, the worksheet prompts you to articulate your desire and to identify obstacles that got in your way—as well as what you did to overcome those obstacles. Your story may include more than one obstacle, and in that case, you can repeat the steps. Obstacles can be physical of course, but they can also be psychological. Not believing you deserve to get what you want can be a far more formidable obstacle than whatever physical one you may have encountered.

— — —

On the last evening of the writing seminar, Sara encouraged me to read to the group what I had feverishly written about Robert the morning after my conversation with her. She said that reading my story first, before any of the other participants shared, would show that I was willing to do what I was asking them to do: be vulnerable. The room that evening was dim, illuminated by a snapping fire on one side of the room and a few floor lamps on the other. The participants and the rest of the seminar staff formed an oval, sitting on antique couches, dusty wingbacks, and creaky wooden chairs.

I read aloud what I had experienced, how it had made me feel, and how I was beginning to see things differently with time and distance. As I had been writing that morning, I realized that I had to commit to seeing Robert as the gift he was, and I had to remind myself that all gifts are temporary. I also thought deeply about how I would support others who were grieving. After being on the receiving end of so many platitudes, I wrote, I decided that I would never again compare or minimize or search for silver linings or grasp at meaning to ennoble the suffering of others. Instead, I promised, I would do what we always try to do at War Horse seminars: show up, bear witness, and grant others the dignity of their own process.

As I approached the climax of the story, I could hear tissues being plucked from boxes and the occasional sniffle. I was afraid that if I looked up from my computer, I'd break into tears as well. When I finished, there was silence at first. Then gentle rubs on my back from those sitting near me. Sara was sitting next to me on the couch. We hugged. Others whispered kind words from across the oval.

Over the next couple hours, nearly all the participants who had spent the past week with me thinking deeply about their stories read their words aloud to the group. As Sara read hers, I felt this sharp sensation, like a slide coming into focus. It was in that moment that I realized something I had always told others was true but had not yet experienced as a writer: stories of trauma and loss and the lessons we pull from them can lead to profound moments of understanding and connectedness when these stories are shared. By the time our gathering dispersed, with the participants feeling lighter than they had all week, I felt an almost primal connection to each of them. And for the first time since my wife and I had lost Robert, I felt like I received the response I had needed all along.

3

Recognizing the Story underneath Your Story

THROUGH THE crack in the bathroom door, I watched my father sob. Raggedly at first. Then unreservedly. He was finally, and maybe for the first time in his life, giving full vent to his emotions. All the frustrations and pent-up anger, all the disappointment and rage. It all drained out of him and onto the linoleum floor. His heart was like a rusty gear that had been frozen for so long that he had forgotten it even existed, until it began to groan and clink along inside his chest. I lingered on the other side of the door, trying not to alert him to my presence. I was transfixed by his grief. It was the first time I can remember seeing him cry.

A few moments later, he took a deep breath and composed himself. It was all too much for me—too private, too confusing. Not wanting to get caught eavesdropping, I darted back into the living room, my heart thumping in my chest as I slumped onto the couch. I swung my legs onto the arm and propped my head up with my right elbow, facing the television, like I hadn't a care in the world, like the sound from the set had covered whatever noise he'd made in the bathroom.

When we learned earlier that day that my grandfather was dead, I didn't think my father would grieve, let alone cry. I thought he'd feel relieved, happy even, that such an awful man was gone. Try as I might that day, I couldn't remember ever hearing a kind word spoken about him. If anything, he was more mythical figure than human, no different from Aesop. Whenever my dad needed to prove to me how much tougher his life had been than mine, he'd tell me a story from his childhood, which was, without question, far worse than his stories could convey. The one that sticks out to me now was one he told me when I was a teenager. A dozen friends of mine were over at our place. It was summertime, and we were stalking through the woods behind my house, playing soldiers and shooting little red paintballs at each other. The brand-new gun I had bought with my birthday money broke less than an hour into the fun, and I was pissed—and acting pissy, I'm sure. To put me in my place, my dad pulled me aside and told me about the prized Holstein he'd raised when he was about my age. His father, quite unexpectedly, let him keep the cash prize from the country fair, which my father used to buy himself a wooden baseball bat. Late one evening, when my father's prize-winning cow stubbornly refused to come back into the barn, my grandfather found the bat and broke it over the cow's head, killing it with a dull thwack. My little *inconvenience*, in comparison, was trivial.

After my father composed himself and left the bathroom, he appeared at the end of the hall that led into our living room. He glanced at me as though he'd forgotten I was home, silently trying to glean how much I knew about what he had been doing. I remember clearly how tired and slumped his face looked. His glasses and goatee hid most of whatever tracks his tears had made. Without saying a word, he turned to his right and stepped down the basement stairs. A few moments later, I heard the television down there come to life. He turned to the same channel I was watching upstairs.

— — —

My father admits that without his high school girlfriend finishing his homework for him, he probably never would have graduated from high school. Academic achievement was good for me—expected even—but it didn't provide him with the same sense of pleasure that he got from watching me crush some kid running the football up the middle under the lights on a Friday night. For as long as I can remember, he's gotten uncomfortable around "smart people" and has dreaded "looking stupid" above nearly all other fears. His father was like that too, I've been told. And when my father was stressed or sleep deprived from the swing shift he worked at the paper mill, he would lose his temper about the strangest, seemingly most insignificant, things. Leaving toothpaste residue on a washcloth or forgetting to replace a pen cap after taking a phone message would suddenly become life-or-death situations that needed immediate rectification. Sometimes he'd break things or put holes in the wall by throwing whatever object he was holding that hadn't performed the way he desired. If he was really angry, he'd storm out of the house and peel out of the driveway in the car like a madman. When he returned, he would meet me or my mother with silence, probably deeply embarrassed by his behavior but unwilling or unable to own up to it and apologize or explain what was really bothering him. It couldn't really have been the toothpaste residue, could it? Instead, he would seclude himself in the basement for days or weeks until none of us could remember exactly what had happened or what he'd been so upset about. Then one day, it would all be over; he just wanted us to forget whatever had happened and go back to pretending everything was fine. The only readily discernable ways he was unlike his now-dead father were that my father didn't drink and didn't beat up on me, my younger brother, or my mother. For that, I am grateful.

By the time I was old enough to remember anything about him, my grandfather had become nothing more than a pathetic, bewildered old man. Some say that after my grandmother, Gladys, left him for another man, my Grandpa Hod mellowed and became much less volatile, more submissive. By that time, however, the damage was done, and in the few years before he died, my grandfather had created so much distance between himself and anyone else that getting to know him in any deep and meaningful way was out of the question. I never ate a meal with him. He never sent me a birthday card or bought me a scoop of ice cream. I have no fond memories of him teaching me to fish or hit a baseball. As far back as I can remember, he was nothing but a tragic, untold story.

After everyone had left him, my grandfather lived alone on the family farm for several years, boarding up most of the bedrooms and other space he didn't use daily. When the bank took it over and sold it to an Amish family, most of the rat-infested interior had to be gutted and replaced. With only what he could pack into the back of a rusted pickup truck, he took what little money he had left and paid cash for a run-down, one-bedroom shack of a house across the street from the Lutheran church in the tiny farming community of Taylor, Wisconsin, only a few blocks away from where my grandmother lived with her second husband, Ray.

Highway 95, which runs along the northern end of town, connects Taylor to a series of small farming communities to the east and west. The sights along the highway between these communities mostly consist of old family farmhouses in dire need of new paint, half-collapsed red barns begging for a match, fenced fields of mud-splattered Guernseys and Holsteins, and woebegone mobile homes parked behind cluttered, overgrown lawns. My father says he can guess what time of year it is around there just by the smell. Fresh manure in the spring. Rustling stalks of corn in the summer. Hay in the fall. Salt and sand and freshly disked loam in the winter. Hemmed on all sides by fields of corn and soybeans, Taylor was my grandfather's place of birth. He spent nearly every day of his life there. He married and helped run a business there. Each of his five children was born there. He would have died there, too, if my father hadn't found him that steaming Friday afternoon in August 2000.

— — —

The first thing I always noticed when we arrived at my grandfather's house for our annual check-in was the battered shell of a rusted-out John Deere tractor rotting in the unmown grass of his front yard. Crumbling concrete steps and a rusty pipe for a handrail led to the front door. When we would visit him, my father would go inside first, leaving us behind in the yard. There was always a hollowness in the air, a dark, unspeakable silence as we waited for my father to return to the steps and give us the go-ahead to enter. I didn't realize it until I was much older, but my father was checking to make sure my grandfather was still alive inside.

Once we got the go-ahead, my mother, brother, and I would file into the kitchen and line up, tallest to shortest. With only one kitchen chair to his name, no one except my grandfather could sit, not that we would have wanted to if there were enough chairs to go around. The stained linoleum floor and the windowsill above his rusty steel, Formica-topped table were layered with dust and dead flies. My grandfather would sit as we stood looking at him, politely hoping not to stick to anything—or pass out from the natural gas slowly leaking from his old stove. I remember trying to ignore it all and fixating on the way he would dig the bloated knuckles of his left hand into the top of his thigh to keep himself propped up. Even though he'd been retired for years, his hands were still calloused, his fingernails lined with grease. His eyes were a deep blue, like mine, and his face was rough and broken in a way that could have been handsome. I remember too his sweet and sour smell of brandy and sweat. He seemed to be locked in a car on a road he didn't want to be on.

My father always did most of the talking, usually about the weather and other such banalities. He seemed so different while in his father's presence. Diminished somehow, hiding behind a carefree demeanor, like all of this was normal or acceptable. As we got older, my father would tell him stories about us kids, our athletic exploits or academic achievements. He would laugh at his own punchlines, trying to dissipate the discomfort that pulled us down like a wet blanket around our shoulders. What memories did my father have to suppress to put on such a charade? The tension was exhausting. Fifteen minutes after we arrived, just before the noxious fumes induced a throbbing headache, my father would make some excuse about why we had to leave.

— —— —

My grandfather died on a Sunday. He was a rough-hewn man, under-educated and overburdened, who fought in World War II and came home a drunk. It didn't seem like he had wanted to fight in the war. Some think that's why he knocked up my grandmother before either one of them could finish high school. Maybe he thought they wouldn't need a man with a baby on the way. The draft board took him anyway, and by the time his daughter was born, in the early fall of 1944, he was training for war. By the time he turned 19, he was on the Japanese island of Okinawa, fighting in the longest and deadliest battle of the Pacific theater. Like many men of his generation, he didn't like to talk about his war. He never spoke a word about it to me, and my father remembers only a handful of stories, fragments really.

I once heard a story about my grandfather from my father's older brother. I was told that when my grandfather was a younger man, when he still hung around some of the other veterans in town, he would talk sometimes. Only to other veterans, though. Usually around the John Deere tractor repair shop my grandfather ran with his father. My uncle would hang around there sometimes when he was little and listen in when the other fellas started telling their stories. He remembers Hod mostly listening while he turned wrenches and checked fluids, sometimes scoffing or rolling his eyes at the stories that were probably closer to tall tales. If someone pressed my grandfather to share something about the war, he would look up from whatever motor he was working on and tell them about the Sherman tanks he was trained to drive, what a pain in the ass they were to steer. He'd laugh about the sergeant he met at the processing center at Fort Sheridan, just north of Chicago, who discovered that my grandfather had grown up on a farm and knew how to drive a tractor. *If you can drive a tractor,* he'd said, *you can drive a tank.* Round peg. Round hole. Sometimes he'd say that his tank company had been nearly wiped out in some disastrous battle no one back home had ever heard about, that the mission was doomed from the beginning. Incompetent officers, he'd say, as he wiped the sweat from his brow with the back of his grease-stained hand. The other vets would nod in commiseration.

I was only 14 years old when my grandfather passed. At that time, I hadn't heard any of these stories about him. I didn't know where he had served or what he had done. I only found those things out later, after I began my investigation. All I knew was that he had fought and that he had come home a changed man. That's what everyone said. In the years after the war, he did things and said things—terrible things. Things no husband or father should ever do or say, things that people avoided talking about because he was a war hero. But I didn't know what those things were exactly. My father's family didn't like to talk about them. My father hated being asked questions about the past. Most of what I learned about my grandfather I learned from my mother when I was a teenager.

— — —

On the day before my grandfather was to be buried, the nondescript funeral home that prepared his body hosted a wake in the early evening. The front entryway smelled like flowers, a nice complement to the scent of freshly cut grass that dominated the air outside. My father and I found my grandfather's silver casket open at the upper half and positioned as far from the door to the parlor as possible. Standing sprays of blue and white flanked each end, and a small oak table with a folded American flag and a black-and-white photo of my grandfather in his service uniform stood sentry near the foot. The funeral director was nowhere to be found, so my father ducked out of the parlor to find him. Left alone with my grandfather, I felt this strange compulsion to see his body up close.

When I reached the foot of his casket, I looked at the framed photo of my grandfather and then peered over the edge at what had become of that young man. The first thing I noticed, after pushing my glasses higher up my nose, was how healthy he looked compared to the last time I'd seen him alive. That time he was lying in a hospital bed, trapped beneath a tangle of cords and tubes. His body was swollen in misery.

He had been near death when my father found him sitting on his kitchen chair, legs spread wide, his bloated gut resting between his thighs and bulging out of his dirty overalls. His breathing was labored; his eyes bulged out of his head. I doubt he had been expecting company. If he had been, he probably would have made sure not to get caught with a half-empty bottle of blackberry brandy and a garbage can full of crushed Old Style beer cans.

The year before, the doctors at the VA told my father that if my grandfather didn't stop drinking, he'd soon be dead. And it wouldn't be quick or painless, either. Cirrhosis of the liver kills slowly. On top of that, my grandfather's blood pressure was way too high, the doctors said, and none of the medications they had tried was having much of an effect. He was also losing excretory function. My father wasn't sure what that meant and at the time didn't have the wherewithal to ask for clarification. Plus, there was his massively bloated belly, not to mention hepatic encephalopathy (buildup of blood-borne toxins in the brain) and renal impairment. That's what you get, the doctors said, after nearly six decades of drowning your pain in liquor.

With my grandfather slumped in the back seat of the car, my father sped to the hospital. He tried to keep him awake and talking about the weather and how the hay was ready for the third harvest of the season. Back when my grandfather worked as a mechanic, this would have been a busy time for him. For four decades, he had been known as the best combine mechanic in three counties; it was the only thing he was ever good at.

At his father's bedside in the hospital, my father wanted to say something—anything. He would have liked to say goodbye and tell his father he forgave him for all the hurt and anguish he had put the family through, but my father couldn't find the words. The shame was still too raw, the smell too intense. He wasn't even dead yet, but my grandfather had begun to rot. Instead of talking, my father stood and stared at this man who had scared and tormented him for so long, who was now nothing more than a weak, dying old man. He looked at his face, the wisps of hair on the top of his head, and the silver three-day-old stubble that covered his chin and cheeks. He saw himself. Unlike the rest of his siblings, my father couldn't bring himself to forgive or even hope that he and his father were going to get another chance, in some other place at some other time, to discover who the other was. He didn't understand his father, and his father didn't understand him, and there was nothing he could say in those last few hours to change that.

Lying in his casket at the funeral home, my grandfather looked peaceful and calm—a testament to the funeral director's skill. The caked-on makeup covered up the evidence of the broken blood vessels, and a clean shave paired with the desiccation that occurs at death left him looking square-jawed and resolute. His eyes and mouth were closed, and his upper body was dressed in a white, short-sleeved, button-up shirt long out of style.

I realized as I came up next to him that I had never really studied his face before. Looking closely at it for the first time, I felt alone with him and scared of what his body might feel like. I pictured him opening his eyes, smiling at me, like this was all some elaborate practical joke. After turning to see whether anyone had entered the parlor without me realizing it, I turned back to my grandfather and reached out a shaking hand. I poked his chest, just under the collarbone. There was no elasticity to his skin. Not like when you poke the jellylike body of a deer you've just shot to make sure it's really dead. He was more rock than flesh. Feeling emboldened, I placed my left hand on his chest, near where his heart once beat. It was only for a moment. Then I heard a rustling behind me and quickly stuffed both my hands into my pockets. I kept looking at my grandfather's face, pretending I hadn't just felt him up, as my father walked up from behind and to my left. He placed his right hand on my left shoulder and stared inside the casket with me.

The dark, yellowy complexion of my grandfather's face made it seem as if it had been sculpted in wax. I realize now, all these years later, that it was this waxiness that prevented any feeling of intimacy, not that there ever had been any of that before he died.

I don't remember crying that day. Maybe because I was no longer looking at my grandfather but rather at something that resembled him. A shell that was once a body. Or maybe because I never really knew him, because he never wanted to be known. As far as I was concerned, he was but a couple of pictures and a handful of fragmented stories. How do you mourn such an abstraction?

— — —

When I was young, I didn't know how to ask about my grandfather. I wanted to know why he lived by himself in a run-down shack with dirty tractor parts piled on the kitchen table and even dirtier dishes stacked in the sink. I wanted to know why he drank so much and didn't take care of himself. I wanted to know why he never came for Christmas or even mailed a birthday card. There were so many unanswered questions. Even as I grew older, I still felt like I couldn't get the answers I needed. His story had become a taboo of sorts, not because it was a secret per se, but because it was unknown and because polite folks didn't talk about those sorts of things where I come from.

What really happened to my grandfather during the war? Something *must* have happened, we all thought. How bad was that tank battle, really? Did his tank survive? Or was it hit, and he had to save himself somehow? Did he lose any friends? Did he ever kill anyone? No one could be sure. None of us knew the details of what he experienced, except for witnessing the mental and emotional damage these things left in their wake.

After I finished graduate school in 2010, I started asking questions again, looking for answers. I was tired of the silence. I was tired of the guessing and the lack of curiosity. The fake acceptance. The fear of acceptance. At that time, I believed my father was avoiding his memories like a man who makes peace with the scars from a car accident he can't bring himself to remember. *It's in the past. Forget it. It doesn't matter now, anyway.* But I couldn't. I'm not like my father, I told myself. I couldn't pretend the past wasn't real. I couldn't accept that we didn't know the truth. I couldn't just walk away from the smoke and the muffled screams of the overturned car in the ditch that was my family's past. I couldn't ignore the blood splattered on the road. I had to search. I had to investigate. I had to make sense of it all.

There's a Story underneath Your Story

By this point in the writing process, we know that in a story needing to be told, the main character has to want something, an "object of desire." And then something else prevents the character from getting the object of desire, so the character struggles against that opposing force and either succeeds or fails. We also know that a story needing to be told will show transformation and growth over time as the result of a conflict. After having read this story about my father and grandfather, what would you say my object of desire was?

If you guessed that I wanted to find out what my grandfather had experienced during World War II, you're exactly right. I didn't understand why my father was so upset when his father died. I had very little understanding of who my grandfather was or what he had survived. I felt like I needed to know to feel whole. Though now I know that's not exactly true. That's my object of desire.

But what about my real *need*?

What was I lacking mentally, emotionally, or spiritually?

What was the story *underneath* my story?

"Every work of literature has both a situation and a story," writes Vivian Gornick, the author of *The Situation and the Story*. "The situation is the context or circumstance, sometimes the plot; the story is the emotional experience that preoccupies the writer: the insight, the wisdom, the thing one has come to say."[1] It has been my experience that the "thing" one has come to say generally relates to some subconscious need the writer simply cannot thrive without.

Think about your story. What did you really *need*? What were you lacking? What did you need to learn or realize in order to disprove a misconception about yourself or the world? More often than not, your subconscious need is nothing more than a realization of some kind of truth. When you finally face that truth, your perspective on yourself or the world around you will be transformed. You will, in turn, be able to deal with whatever problems life throws at you. There are several needs harbored by nearly every human being on the planet, including the need to

- accept reality,
- forgive or be forgiven,
- overcome fear,
- find courage,
- nurture faith in oneself and in others,
- nurture faith in a higher power,
- love and be loved,
- trust and be trusted,
- overcome the power of greed,
- stand up for something one believes in,
- do one's duty,
- atone, and
- survive.

Many writers, once they uncover that need, come right out and tell the reader exactly what the story underneath the story is. Other writers, of course, tell personal stories that are subtler and leave room for the reader to interpret. That's a matter of style, and you can approach your story whichever way makes more sense for you.

— — —

I have always been a perfectionist who has done things passionately and lived intensely in new interests. And when whatever passion I had was suddenly spent, everything associated with it got thrown into a box: playing football and the guitar, bowhunting and throwing ceramic pots and painting, triathlons and German history. Every time I moved—from Stevens Point, Wisconsin, to Chicago for graduate school; from Chicago to Washington, DC, for work; and from DC back to Wisconsin for Ashley's career—those boxes were sold at garage sales, dropped off at Goodwill, or left next to sticky green dumpsters behind apartment buildings. Moving on from a previous passion was what I had to do to make room for the next one. That's how it was with all things related to my father, too.

When I was growing up, being his son was like a full-time job that took nearly everything I had. When I left home for college, our relationship was more like a part-time job. The hours weren't great. The pay was insulting, and it was difficult for me to see how it was ever going to help get me where I needed to go. Until my father and I started our journey to uncover the truth about what happened to my grandfather during the Battle of Okinawa, my relationship with him had morphed into something closer to a hobby, something I once engaged in passionately but had since collected dust in the back of a closet.

What Kind of Story Are You Trying to Tell?

In a seminal article published in 1955, Norman Friedman named, defined, and illustrated 14 types of stories he believed all literary works are shaped by. Of the 14 types of stories he laid out, there are four that I commonly see when working with trauma survivors. The first type, which Friedman called *maturing* stories, involves a sympathetic main character "whose goals are either mistakenly conceived or undermined and whose will is consequently rudderless and vacillating."[2] The cause for such a condition is inexperience and naïveté. By the end of a maturing story, the main character must find strength and direction, "and this may be accomplished through some drastic, or even fatal, misfortune," Friedman continued. In the end, what makes for a satisfactory ending to a maturing story is the "crucial element of choice, of coming finally to a radical decision."[3]

Of all the types of stories Friedman laid out in his article, what he called *education* stories are, in my experience, by far the most common among trauma survivors. Education stories involve a "change in thought for the better" in the main character's conceptions, beliefs, and attitudes. Similar to a maturing story, the main character's way of seeing the world at the beginning of an education story is somehow inadequate and is changed for the better—a change in the direction of "a more comprehensive view" of the world. Main characters in maturing or education stories, Friedman wrote, undergo a threat of some sort and emerge "into a new and better kind of wholeness at the end, with a final sense of relief, satisfaction, and pleasure."[4]

Put another way, the main character in an education or maturing story must change by overcoming something within themselves, usually by giving up something they *want* in order to get what they really *need*. Think back to the story I included in chapter 2 about losing my son. What I wanted was him. What I needed, however, was to learn how to grieve and accept what I cannot change. That's a shift in my view of life from a naïve, largely uninformed perspective to a new and more mature and meaningful one. If I had to sum up the story underneath the story of losing my son, I'd say this: wisdom conquered my depression when I learned to accept the world as paradoxical and imperfect.

If you're interested in writing such a story, be mindful that your readers will want to know what you knew at the beginning, what you believed, and how you saw the world. Something in that state of things needs to change. Did you accept the truth presented to you, or did you continue to cling to your beliefs until the very end? The point of the story isn't to educate the reader exactly but rather to show the reader how meaning is gained when we finally learn to express ourselves or make sense of the lessons we've learned.

There are also what Friedman called *disillusionment* stories, which involve a sympathetic main character who "starts out in the full bloom of faith in a certain set of ideals." After being subjected to some sort of loss, threat, or trial, Friedman continued, the main character "loses faith entirely." Such a story usually ends with the main character resembling a "puppet without wires or a clock with a broken mainspring." Fear overcomes hope, and the reader is usually left with a sense of loss and even pity.[5] If done well, disillusionment stories can be instructive for a reader by shining a light on experiences that are oftentimes viewed as ennobling (loss, struggle, trauma, and grief) but are far more complicated than is commonly acknowledged.

I usually steer writers away from disillusionment stories unless their explicit goal is to elicit a feeling of loss or pity in their readers. That's how most readers tend to react to stories that do not end with a more positive resolution. Whereas maturing stories are about accepting the paradoxical and imperfect nature of life on planet Earth, disillusionment stories are essentially about refusing to accept this.

The fourth type of story I often see is what Friedman called *degeneration* stories. In such a story, the main character we meet at the beginning is sympathetic and full of ambition but, through the course of the story, is subjected to "some crucial loss which results in his utter disillusionment." The main character, Friedman continues, then "has to choose between picking up the threads of his life and starting over again, or giving up his goals and ambitions altogether."[6]

There's one other kind of story I commonly see—and sometimes write. In what I call a *revelation* story, the main character transforms from a state of ignorance to a state of knowledge through the revelation of previously unknown information. More specifically, the main character in a revelation story lacks essential facts, has doubt about their circumstances that leads to a revelation or to a shocking truth, and makes wise and appropriate decisions in response. The story of my journey to uncover the truth about what my grandfather experienced in World War II, which weaves its way through much of this book, is the best example I have of a revelation story. The payoff for the reader is either a state of relief or satisfaction when the main character learns something essential or pity and horror when the main character finds out the truth only after it's too late.

— — — — — —

In the late summer of 2012, Ashley and I decided to move our growing family back to Wisconsin. At the time, I was working as a communications specialist at the US Government Accountability Office in Washington, DC. The Government Accountability Office has a small field office in downtown Chicago, near the train station that could take me to and from Kenosha, where my wife grew up, just over the Illinois-Wisconsin border. We thought we could probably afford a small house in Kenosha and that childcare would be cheaper, too. In DC, what money I made while Ashley was finishing her unpaid internship in dietetics was spent almost entirely on our rent and our son's daycare bill. Whatever we spent on food or clothes or entertainment came out of what little savings we had left from our wedding two summers before.

In early August, a few weeks before our apartment lease expired, Ashley and our son, George, flew from DC to Wisconsin so that Ashley could start working her new job at the Cancer Treatment Centers of America. Money was going to be tight—I wasn't even sure my check for the moving truck was going to clear—and we were going to need whatever we could get as soon as we could get it.

When I told my father about my plan to drive the moving truck back to Wisconsin on my own, he rejected that idea as nonsense and said he'd take some time off and fly out to help me pack and keep me company on the long drive across the country. After he and I finished loading the truck, the night before we planned to hit the road, we took the Metro's red line into the district to see the monuments on the National Mall lit up with floodlights. I didn't know it when we left, but he had taken all the research I had been doing on my grandfather and registered Hod in the National World War II Memorial Registry. He wanted to look it up on one of the kiosks located just south of the National World War II Memorial, which lies midway between the Washington Monument and the Lincoln Memorial.

The World War II Memorial is grand and oval shaped. Very clean. At the south end is an arch labeled "Pacific." To the north is the Atlantic arch. Stone pillars, adorned with green copper wreaths, stand along the oval's periphery—one pillar for each state and US territory. In the center of the west side of the monument is a low wall on which 4,048 gold metal stars are pinned. One for every thousand American troops who were killed during World War II: 405,399 souls. Twelve of those stars represent the 12,000 Americans who lost their lives in the Battle of Okinawa. "Here we mark the price of freedom," reads a sign in front of the wall. I wish I could say I care for war monuments. I have an especially hard time with the World War II Memorial. It's too symmetrical, too orderly. If there's one thing I've learned from all the research I've done, it's that World War II was none of those things.

Standing at the registry's kiosk, after typing in my grandfather's last name and hometown, we saw his name pop up on the screen. My father looked relieved. He turned and smiled at me. "There he is," he said.

On our walk back to the Metro station, my father kept talking. "After all the research you've done," he said, "and everything you've found, it's really made me think. I wish I could say it has made me forgive him, but it hasn't."

"I understand," I said as the train approached the dimly lit train platform.

"But I feel like," he said, "I feel like I better understand him."

— —— —

We began a 17-hour drive to Wisconsin via Interstate 80 the next morning. Because we were going to be trapped in the cab of a yellow Penske moving truck for all that time, I decided to finally ask him all the questions I had always wanted answers to. He seemed ready to have this conversation with me and laid out the timeline of his life without much coaxing. He told me more about his childhood and his early adolescence, about his time in the Army and his shotgun marriage to my half-sister's mother. He told me stories of my mother, from before I was born, and what he remembered of me from when I was George's age. For the first time, I felt like I had known who my father was and who he had wanted to be. He had never confided in me like that before, and I soaked up as much as I could, putting together the pieces of the puzzle in my mind. When he told me more about being a father, his cheeks reddened, and his posture become more erect. My heart twitched like a dreaming dog. He hadn't been a very good father, he admitted. But he had done the best he could—much better than his own father ever did, he added. And look at how I had turned out, he said; I had a graduate degree and a beautiful family. While he regretted much of what he had done—and even more of what he hadn't done—he had nothing more to give.

His arms were crossed in the passenger seat, and his left hand was stroking his graying goatee. He didn't say anything for a long time. I couldn't tell if he was lost in thought or waiting for me to reply. Then he told me more about his own father. He said that my grandfather's father, Harry, was the only person my grandfather seemed to be able to talk to, the only person who had any sort of influence over him. Harry was a short and sinewy man who could hammer nails with both hands at the same time and who could run circles around anyone else in town, even though he had only one lung. He had one of his lungs removed after breathing in too much dust while working at a feed mill. When my grandfather's behavior got too out of hand—like the time he shoved a shotgun in my grandmother's face after she refused to come home and subject herself and her children to his tirades—it was Harry who was able to talk some sense into my grandfather, which made things better, at least for a little while.

By the time my father was old enough to really get to know his grandfather, Harry died from a massive heart attack. That was in the spring of 1971. Four months later, my father's oldest sister, Charlene, passed away as well. She had been living in a mental institution and died from an infection. The state had placed her in the institution after she fell and hit her head on the kitchen counter at the age of nine. Her brain had swelled, and she developed epilepsy and never progressed cognitively past the level of a small child. My father said that the family visited her only a couple times per year, usually on her birthday and around Christmas time, and that she never knew who they were or why they were there to visit her. My aunt Mary told me once that my grandmother never forgave herself for letting my grandfather talk her into letting the state take Charlene way.

After Harry and Charlene passed, "That's when he went really downhill," my father said. "Still a hard worker—always worked hard. But he drank more, took care of himself less. I saw him break down once. We went to bail some hay, and Dad broke down, weeping. Said he missed his father. That was the only time I ever saw him cry."

Whatever anger and bitterness he felt about losing his father and daughter, he projected onto my grandmother and the rest of his kids, which only deepened the wounds of his marriage. With his restless demands, emotional stinginess, detachment, and unprovoked bursts of violence, my grandfather became nearly impossible to live with. After work, he would stop at the bar, knock back a few, and then, with darkness falling, he'd roar home to do chores. After downing more booze in the barn, he'd burst into the house, demanding his supper be ready that instant. The family lived in constant fear of him. His rampages could swerve in any direction.

"He was very abusive, just mean," my father told me. "Called Mom names, always bitching about everything. Mad about the government and what he had to do in World War II. What they promised and never paid up. Nothing was his fault."

"Did he ever apologize? Or even feel bad the next day?" I asked.

My father thought for a moment. "No," he said. He paused again. "I don't remember him ever apologizing. He never tried to make amends. He would just pretend it had never happened. Sometimes he would blame Mom."

"You know," he continued, "he actually seemed to enjoy making us feel shitty. He did things to me—said things, too—that hurt so badly. He would stick his rubber boots in the barn gutter with the shit and all that and then kick me in the ass. Backhanded me a lot. He always had something mean to say. As I got older, I tried to distract him and take the brunt of whatever it was that pissed him off so much. That way Mom wouldn't have to keep taking it as much."

Things grew so bad that Harry's business partner refused to partner with my grandfather after Harry's death and instead bought my grandfather out of the John Deere repair business. He agreed to keep my grandfather on as chief mechanic, but the damage to my grandfather's pride never scabbed over. A couple of years later, in the winter of my father's senior year of high school, my grandfather threw him out of the house after my father tried to protect my grandmother from one of his drunken punch fests. The sting of being cast out and rejected by his own father cut deeply. I'm not convinced my father has ever gotten over it.

After stopping for gas and checking the tow straps holding my Oldsmobile tight to the trailer we were hauling, my father seemed eager to keep talking. "Do you know if Grandpa Hod ever talked to anyone about Okinawa?" I asked after climbing back into the driver's seat.

My father thought for a moment, his hand cupping his chin. "Yeah," he said. "There was one." He seemed to feel relieved to field a question unrelated to himself. "Bob Mingus was with the 101st Airborne in Vietnam. Him and his wife, who he had met at a New Jersey VA center, moved to our area, and he was on total disability for emotional problems pertaining to the Vietnam War. He and Dad got along real well. They just connected." He moved his hands side to side like he was holding a basketball and trying to juke a defender. "They just understood each other."

"Did he ever tell you about anything him and your Dad talked about?" I asked.

He chuckled. "Ya know, he talked to me after Dad's funeral. He said, 'I just want to tell you that your dad killed a sniper over in Okinawa.'" His impression of Bob's voice made Bob sound like a bit of a loon. "Whether he did or not—or whether that was just Bob's way . . ."

"Trying to make you feel better?" I interjected.

"Yeah." He paused again. There was a peculiar detachment in his voice, as if he was withdrawn from his words. "Yeah . . . so . . . it wouldn't surprise me." With his right index finger, he rubbed the skin under his right eye. He seemed to be back somewhere else. Then he was back with me. He adjusted his glasses, took a deep breath. "There were lots of snipers over there, so who knows?" He chuckled.

"He was feared," my father continued, "but he was well liked. Even sometimes in the bar, there'd be a certain mood every once in a while where I think the young Hod came out, where he was almost like the center of attention, and he was full of life and laughing and having a good time with people and playing cards, but those times were few and far between." He adjusted his baseball cap, snugging it down on his head, shaking the brim side to side before finding the right spot. "Most other times, he was very stoic, drinking his drink. The years went by, and he'd talk to some people, but just . . ." My father was beginning to seem resigned, like he was tiring of our talk and waiting for me to move on to some other topic. "Then he'd have his fill and go home."

"Ya know," he continued a little while later, "I never, basically I never learned anything from him. Never sat me down and taught me how to be a mechanic, work with wrenches. Even to farm; he never taught me how to plant corn, plant oats, or things like that. He just never taught me anything, and I never really learned anything from him." His face was drawn in an expression of intense suffering. Then, for a moment, he lost all interest in what he was talking about and uncoiled like a spring. "The only thing he ever really gave me was that rusted old John Deere, that Model B he had parked in his yard—you remember when I had that restored?"

"Yeah, of course," I replied. I had wanted my father to keep it until I had a garage big enough to store it, but the prohibitive cost of a monthly storage unit forced him to sell it to some collector from Iowa.

"He never got to see it in person again, just pictures of it all fixed up. He was impressed with what I did," my father said. "And when you think about it, he was a mechanic, and he took this running tractor and parked it in the yard and let it turn into a bucket of rusted bolts with a frozen engine and rotted tires, which is basically how my life was living with him." He chuckled again, but not because he was happy. He was trying to defuse the emotional response he was having to the memories of his childhood. "He was a good man," my father continued, "in so many ways, but . . ." He couldn't find the words. "For whatever reason, when he reached that certain period when his old man and Charlene, and the business, and all that went away—I call it the 'social drinker turning into the hard alcoholic'—he just stopped taking care of himself, and he didn't seem to care about what people thought about him."

"He became a rusted bucket of bolts," I said.

"Yep. He was. And I'm not embarrassed to say it, but he embarrassed me."

"He didn't live up to whatever ideal there was for the Greatest Generation," I said.

"No, not at all. He became one of the town drunks, and most of the time, even in the wintertime, I would walk to and from basketball practice or whatever, just so he wasn't dropping me off. He was embarrassing." He thought for a moment. "Not sure if I ever told you, but Jerry, my older brother, rolled our family's 1950 Chevrolet Deluxe drag racing it in 1964. Dad got in there, laid on his back across the seats, and pushed the roof back up. And it was all dented and scratched from rolling down a hill, and the top was crumpled. He drove that for five more years. That was our family vehicle. And then . . ." He lifted his hands in the air, level with his ears, arms straight out, exasperated. "He buys a 1964 Chevy pickup with a Ford back end. That was a laughing matter for everybody. A few times when I would drive with him on a call out into the county to work on a piece of equipment, he would stop at these country stores that were all over the place outside town—a place for the area farmers to pick stuff up—and he'd pick up a six-pack. He'd drink three beers on the way to the farmer who needed his help and drink three more on the way back to the shop. Every call he went on—same thing. He was very embarrassing, which, I don't know, is probably why I get so damn embarrassed when I do stupid things. In a lot of ways, I just feel like I was never shown much of a life."

He moved his arms back and forth from his body, like he was trying to gather supplies off a table. "I didn't know how to . . . go out and get something. I don't know. Just never experienced that." He seemed as though he just realized that I had dissected him, cut into him with a knife and opened him up. His misery was revealed, and I had led him to it.

"I'm sorry that happened to you," I said. It felt like all the other times I'd said those words—for things I both was and was not sorry for. He nodded, uncomfortable with my attempt at empathy. The air between us became still, like a wall. In the silence that followed, I could feel the past crawling over him like lice, laying eggs and colonizing.

The little boy in me wanted to tell him how it had been for me in his absence, but I decided not to go there. I sensed that was a path to a place of hurt feelings from which we'd both leave feeling completely misunderstood. I had no more questions. Silence filled the truck cabin. After a while, I tuned the radio to the 2012 Republican National Convention on public radio. For most of the rest of our time on the highway that night, we talked history and politics, two things we could always discuss and nearly always agreed on.

References

1. Vivian Gornick, *The Situation and the Story: The Art of Personal Narrative* (New York: Farrar, Straus and Giroux), 13.
2. Norman Friedman, "Forms of the Plot," *Journal of General Education* 8, no. 4 (July 1955): 249.
3. Friedman, "Forms of the Plot," 250.
4. Friedman, "Forms of the Plot," 251.
5. Friedman, "Forms of the Plot," 252.
6. Friedman, "Forms of the Plot," 250–51.

| 4 |

Turning Yourself into a Character

I FOUND A deal online that included flights to and from Okinawa and a stay at a nice resort, right on the ocean, over Memorial Day weekend in 2016. I knew my father wouldn't come if he had to rough it or stay somewhere without air conditioning. After working 30 years in a steamy paper mill, he understandably had no interest in suffering heat outside work, too. I also arranged for us to be chauffeured around the island by an old high school classmate of mine, Sarah, who had married a Marine who was stationed on the island. The real clincher, though, was that I found an amateur battlefield historian named Jack Letscher, who agreed to take me and my father to the actual sites of the battles my grandfather's tank company had fought.

When I called my father to tell him about the trip and said he didn't have to worry about paying for a thing, he fell silent. I was surprised. I had built up this moment in my mind where he'd excitedly accept my invitation or maybe even fight back tears of joy at the thought of us finally putting to rest, together, whatever still weighed so heavily on him.

When he refused to come along, I wasn't so much shocked as dismayed. He told me he had no interest in burning vacation time to travel to an "armpit of the world." What he didn't tell me on that call was that he was scheduled to undergo a complicated heart procedure to correct an atrial fibrillation six weeks before Memorial Day and that he wasn't sure he'd be recovered by the time I wanted to go to Okinawa. He also never told me that he wasn't so sure he was even going to make it off the operating table.

Sue, my father's wife, called me a few days before the surgery. She said my father hadn't told me about it because he didn't want to worry me, but she needed me to come to the hospital because there was a distinct possibility I might be needed. "For what?" I asked her. I thought she meant for comfort or support, which seemed odd. That's not the kind of relationship my father and I had. "The surgeon says your father could throw a clot during the ablation procedure," Sue said, "and they wouldn't know if that has happened until after the anesthesia wears off. If that does happen, they may need a relative who can donate blood. The surgeon says an adult child is best."

Sue said I needed to be there at 5:30 a.m. on Wednesday. I canceled my classes and called in sick to my government job. My father's older sister, Mary, offered to drive me to the hospital because she wanted to be there, too.

My father seemed happy to have me at the hospital the next morning. His central line had already been placed, and he was naked beneath his hospital gown. When I asked him why he hadn't wanted to tell me about the procedure at first, he said he didn't want to worry me or put me out; he knew I was busy with family, work, and travel.

He used to be amused that I divided my time among several places: my Tudor Revival across the street from the university where I taught nearly full-time; my in-laws' mellow Cape Cod in Kenosha, where I stayed when I needed to travel every other week to Chicago for my government job; the Grand Hyatt in Washington, DC, near the headquarters building of the Government Accountability Office; and various hotel and motel rooms—whatever was cheapest—across the country wherever there was a university or community college that wanted me to speak about my work and the lessons I'd learned by teaching student veterans how to tell their stories of service, war, and coming home. Sometimes it felt like my home in Wisconsin was little more than a pit stop between trips.

"You're always on the road," he lamented once during one of our infrequent phone conversations, right after we'd finished complaining about the Republicans in Congress and before we awkwardly said we loved each other just before hanging up. "I know, Dad. I know," I said. "Someday it's all going to pay off." I pictured him shaking his head in silent bewilderment on the other end of the line. If he could have had his way, he'd probably still be living in the single-story ranch house I grew up in on Woodland Drive. He loved that house. My mother didn't. It was too small. She wanted an oasis, someplace to make her art and enjoy the beauty of northern Wisconsin.

When I was a freshman in high school, not long after my grandfather passed, my mother decided it was time to move into a bigger, grander house. The newly constructed home my parents bought on six acres of land 10 miles outside town had all the character she was looking for but also turned out to have 157 code violations. A structural engineer they hired to evaluate it after we moved in said he could collapse it that afternoon if we wanted him to. The stress of the resulting lawsuit was too much for my parents' already fragile marriage to endure, and just after I got my driver's license, they decided to call it quits. My brother and I moved with my mother back into town, into a house once owned by my chemistry teacher. My father stayed in the house he hated while it was gutted to the studs and rehabbed back into livable condition. Sometimes he'd lie to himself. He'd think, *One day I'll get over this.* He'd think, *Tomorrow it will be less painful.* Then he'd adjust his glasses and crack his knuckles, and another day would be gone.

When the construction company tasked with the remodeling finished its work, the house sold quickly, and my father moved into a one-bedroom apartment above my mother's best friend's garage a block from the high school. Before too long—and before my parents' divorce was even finalized—my father fell in with a long-divorced woman named Sue, who lived on Woodland Drive half a mile from our old house. He moved in with her, divorced my mother, got married in an intimate ceremony in Central Park that my brother and I were not invited to, and resolved to live a quiet, circumspect life on the street he loved.

A final update from the doctor vibrated Sue's phone several hours after my father's procedure had begun. She pulled her phone from her pocket and announced that my father seemed to be out of danger. "The surgeon says, 'Time will tell if the procedure was a success.'" She broke into silent tears of joy. My aunt Mary hugged her. They stood like that for a long time. I stood with my hands in my pockets, ready for all of it to be over with.

Once he came out from under the anesthesia, and his doctor convinced us that all was well, I told my father that I was glad he was all right but that I was exhausted and needed to get home. That was partly true. The part I didn't tell him was that it was too painful for me to see him trapped beneath a web of cords and tubes, looking so pathetic and old in that recovery room. The image reminded me of my grandfather. On top of all that was happening with my father, his medical issues and our clearly dysfunctional relationship, I felt totally overwhelmed by a number of other challenges, both personal and professional, including a formerly homeless and suicidal vet of the Afghan war who was late, again, on his rent for a small house I was renting to him, a house that he and his black Lab were slowly destroying. My wife and I were also trying for a third baby, though she had recently had a miscarriage and was blaming herself. Then there was the unsustainable balance I had struck at work, where I was working full-time from home for the government and teaching nearly full-time to make ends meet while Ashley finished her master's, all while raising two small boys and trying to maintain a large old house that was in constant need of attention. It was all too much. I felt powerless and paralyzed. Most days I was alone in all of it. I didn't know what to do.

Instead of hanging around the hospital for a second longer than I needed to, I asked my aunt to drop me off at home. I slid my shoes off near the back door and climbed up the steps and into the kitchen. My phone vibrated in my pocket. I ignored it and poured myself four fingers of Balvenie 12-year-old scotch, hoping to be day drunk before Ashley and the kids came home. Just as I took the first sip of that oaky-flavored booze, I checked my phone. A text from Brian Castner. "What are you doing the end of June?" he asked.

"Nothing on the calendar yet," I typed quickly with my free hand. "What's up?"

"Do you want to paddle with me through part of northern Canada? (Nearly) all expenses paid? 10 days?"

"Fuck yeah! Are you kidding?" I typed back.

"Not kidding. I'm still trying to plan this trip down the Mackenzie for book #3. I told you about it, right?"

"Yeah. Count me in."

The Mackenzie River is one of the longest rivers in the world. In 1789, a Scottish fur trader named Alexander Mackenzie, along with a Chipewyan guide named Awgeenah—the "English Chief"—and a handful of voyageurs, their wives, and a few hunters, set out in canoes on the massive waterway in search of the fabled Northwest Passage. Brian was going to paddle the whole damn thing, and he wanted me to paddle one leg of it with him.

"Do you need to ask the boss?" he asked. "Or are you good?"

I hadn't even thought about asking Ashley. I rarely asked her permission for anything. I didn't ask her if a debt-laden yet promising student of mine could move into our basement six months after our second child was born. I didn't ask her if she thought it was a good idea to rent a house to a man we knew had a tendency to cross boundaries and manipulate others for his own personal gain. I hadn't asked her if I could train for and run a 50-mile ultramarathon with Brett. These other people needed me, I told myself. I could help them. I could save them. Why should I ask for permission to do the right thing? And now it was Brian who needed me; there was something so divinely serendipitous about the timing of his text. All other considerations and obligations seemed to melt away like the lone ice cube in my drink.

"Right," I said. "I should probably do that."

— — —

I'm willing to bet you probably don't know much about Brian Castner. Unless you've read one of his books, seen him at a writer's conference, served with him in the Air Force, bumped into him in Buffalo, or Googled him, you probably have no idea what he looks like, sounds like, or what kind of person he is, either. It's not your fault because so far I haven't given you nearly enough information to conjure an image or form an opinion one way or the other. Not to worry, though. I promise that by the end of this chapter, you will see how writers go about turning themselves and others into characters and why it's so important they do so.

On the day Brian invited me to join him on his trip, I wouldn't have said we were friends, exactly. The time we'd be spending on the river would be the longest amount of time we'd ever spent together. Because of the late notice, it was clear that I wasn't his first choice of paddling partner. In our first phone conversation about the trip, he seemed like a relieved, albeit anxious, event planner who books a last-minute replacement for a headlining act. This was no ordinary trip that could easily be postponed or altered in any significant way. He was under contract with a big commercial publisher, and the deadline for his first draft was looming. There were only so many days on the calendar suitable to canoeing the 1,000-plus miles Brian had to cover to reach the Arctic Ocean.

The fact that I wasn't Brian's first choice didn't bother me much. I took his invitation for what it was—an extraordinary opportunity not only to spend two weeks with a man I greatly admired and secretly wanted to be but also to briefly escape what had become of my life. After six years of toiling in what I saw as a dead-end job of writing and editing policy reports and testimonies for a government agency that neither excited nor inspired me in any sustaining way, my life bore little resemblance to what I had once imagined for myself. I felt a vague and inescapable uneasiness on both a spiritual and philosophical level. On paper, my job with the government was enviable, especially considering that I landed it in the summer of 2010, when most of my graduate school classmates were struggling to find anything for which they weren't overqualified. My three closest friends, in fact, had spent the first several years after graduation planning events at the Swedish embassy in Washington, DC, blogging without pay about Soviet utopian architecture, and coaching tennis at an all-boys prep school in St. Louis, respectively. Still, writing reports about the Bureau of Indian Affairs failing to maintain its schools properly on tribal lands or about the exorbitant fees that financial institutions were charging to manage large 401(k) plans wasn't especially challenging for me, and I was routinely turned away when I sought work I felt would have been more fulfilling.

The truth is that I wanted to be like Brian. I didn't want a job or even a career. I wanted a calling. I wanted to feel passionate about my work and to integrate it into my life, to make it a core part of my identity. I wanted to find a literary agent who believed in the story I needed to tell about the military history of my family and the ways in which war trauma radiates through the generations of a family, like a tossed pebble sends ripples across a pond. I wanted my agent to find a big New York publisher, just as Brian's agent had done, that would clamor to cut me a big check for my work. I wanted to connect with my readers, to travel the country reading my words and listening to the stories of folks who could relate to what I had experienced. I wanted to achieve a kind of temporary, two-bit celebrity. I wanted someone, someday, to reach out to me and tell me how much they loved my work. And I wanted someday to text that same person and ask whether they wanted to come on an adventure with me. Most of all, I didn't want to feel like a victim of circumstances, and I wanted Brian to show me the way out of my discontent. That seemed like a fair trade to me: my brawn and my time for his wisdom and a few secrets of the trade.

— — —

At half past seven o'clock on our second day on the water, I awoke to the sound of hundreds of mosquitos hovering near the zippered door of the tent. My neck and cheeks were itchy with swollen bites, and when I slapped a mosquito that had landed on my ankle, blood squirted out onto the yellow interior of Brian's brand-new tent. "The same kind used by climbers on Everest," he had said. Where there was a stiff breeze, the mosquitos were tolerable. On a calm morning, however, they came out in force and blanketed us the instant we emerged into the fresh air. "We're going to hit the actual river today," Brian said as he boiled water for oatmeal and black tea. "Once we find the current, our pace will pick up significantly. Still, we'll need to make up some miles today."

Fourteen hours and 40 miles later, we were ready to set up camp. Our guidebook said there was good camping near the delta of the Kakisa River, a major tributary that drains into the Mackenzie. If there was any good camping there, we didn't see it. Perhaps it was buried somewhere behind the swampy shores of tall grass and weeds that sometimes extended 100 yards or more into the water. It was almost ten o'clock, though I wouldn't have been able to tell it by the sun, which was still a finger or two above the horizon line and radiating orange. Perhaps sensing my dispiritedness, Brian called back to me: "It's going to suck," he said, "but all we can do is keep going until we find something."

Ninety minutes later, we were still floating along the southern shore, our prospects of finding dry earth seeming more and more unlikely by the minute. Wanting to look over the more detailed topographic maps he had rolled into a cardboard tube, Brian told me to steer the canoe up to a shallow spot along the shore where we could get out and stretch our legs. My knees and hips were screaming; they creaked and moaned like an old door as I carefully stepped out of the canoe and into the knee-high water. It took a moment for my back to straighten; my hips still felt tilted forward, unable to realign after being crooked like a question mark for almost 16 hours. Energy poured from my body and dissipated into the water or blew away in the cool breeze. My breathing was starting to quicken. I knew from my time in wilderness first aid that this was a bad sign, so I forced myself to take a deep breath, from the belly, to stave off the panic.

Brian ran his finger on the rolled-out map along the southern edge of the river, from Beaver Lake to a place called Burnt Point. "It looks like there could be good camping here," he said. The rest of the shoreline between where we stood and Burnt Point was labeled "swamp." It was nearly midnight, we were 4,000 miles from home, and it would take another four hours of hard paddling to reach a place that looked like it could have good camping. We were not paddling a designated route in a national wilderness area. There were no park rangers who would come to our rescue, and there was no guarantee that Burnt Point would be anything more than what we'd been paddling past all day. I felt a brutal, self-lacerating despair begin to set in as an even stiffer, cooler breeze picked up. Then my teeth began to chatter; my body shook in waves as I bent down to firm up my grip on the gunnel of the canoe.

"Let's keep paddling and warm you up," Brian said as he rolled up the map.

"You know, we might not find anywhere," I said, my teeth chattering hard enough to hear from the front of the canoe. "What do we do then?"

"We keep going," he said. "We're tired, but we've both been through worse. At least it won't get dark." He was right about that. The night before, the late-June sun had merely skipped across the Arctic tree line before rising once again.

I was physically beat, nearly numb with exhaustion, and circling the top of an abyss, the bottom of which was total collapse of the mind and body. I had no choice about whether I wanted to keep paddling or not.

Halfway to the spot where Brian thought we might find good camping, I spotted an area of dry earth beneath a line of brush. "Is that something?" I said, pointing my canoe paddle to the shore.

"Where?" Brian asked, scanning the shoreline. "Oh, I see it. Right there, right?" he said, pointing his beautiful, custom-made paddle.

My hopes were confirmed, and my sense of doom dissipated, as the Kevlar bottom of our canoe crunched to a halt on a meager stretch of muddy shore. There was just enough dry ground past the nose of the canoe for us to pitch the tent.

"This is perfect," Brian said to my great relief.

Helping Your Readers Picture Your Characters

By this point in the story, you might be trying to picture Brian tying off the canoe on the sturdy base of a shrub hundreds of miles from any semblance of civilization. Perhaps you can see me unloading only the essential gear, rolling out the tent, and assembling the fiberglass tent poles—the camp chores warming my blood, with the midnight sun grazing the tops of the trees to the west. Perhaps in your mind's eye you can picture us crawling into the tent, one after the other, with our sleeping bags under our arms and the bags under our eyes heavy and dark.

What does Brian look like, exactly? What do you know about him? Do you know enough to conjure an image of him? Other than the fact that Brian is a writer and an experienced outdoorsman, what else do you know about him? Not much, right?

Unless you Googled him, you wouldn't know that he has rounded, bearded cheeks, short brown hair, and wears thin-framed glasses. You wouldn't know that he has an average height and build. And unless you met him in person or watched a video of him giving a talk on YouTube, you wouldn't know that he laughs from his chest by sucking in breath as he chuckles when he's nervous or feels awkward.

A quick search online would also tell you that before he became an author, Brian served as an explosive ordnance disposal (EOD) officer in the US Air Force. Unlike many of the men and women he commanded after 9/11, he didn't sign up in a fit of patriotic fervor. Brian wanted to study electrical engineering at Marquette University in Milwaukee, and he received an ROTC scholarship to pay for it. When the Twin Towers crumbled, he was training in Saudi Arabia, counting the days until his required service was complete.

Everything changed, of course, after 9/11, and before his time in the Air Force ended, Brian would deploy twice to Iraq to defuse and clean up the IEDs that littered battlefields afterward. Contrary to what was depicted in *The Hurt Locker*, EOD officers are not reckless adrenaline junkies with a death wish. They are careful and methodical, exacting and analytical. If anyone other than Brian had asked me to paddle 350 miles of wild river thousands of miles from home, I likely would have said no. But I trusted him. He is measured, averse to risk by nature and by training, yet savvy and precise—a two-is-one-and-one-is-none type of planner who believes it's better to be safe than sorry and who can be disarming in his cleverness. He brought all his men home safe from war, and I knew he'd make sure nothing happened to me either.

There are other things about Brian you may or may not need to know. His skin is fair, just like mine, and sunburns easily. Both of us had to goop up with sunscreen constantly and cover as much skin as possible to avoid blistering sunburns. He doesn't really like talking about ideas he has for books. And even though he's a nonfiction writer who takes his craft incredibly seriously, Brian mostly tries to avoid reading other nonfiction books, unless it's for research or if they're about adventure or exploration. He prefers to read novels—Dennis Johnson's *Tree of Smoke* is one of his favorites—and he has an idea for a novel all plotted out, though he would likely never want to speak to me again if I told you any more about it.

— — —

Brian and I first saw Fort Providence's white steeple from about an hour's paddle away. It was nice to have something in the distance to paddle toward, something to break up the monotony of water, shore, and pines. When we reached the town's public boat launch, at the bottom of a hill next to the steeple, Brian studied his GPS and announced that we'd paddled 27 miles that day. After securing our most precious possessions—our money, passports, and electronics—in a small pack Brian would carry on his back, we hiked up the hill and headed east toward the center of town. "If there's a restaurant," Brian said, "I'll buy you a burger and a beer."

Most of the locals we came across on our search for sustenance were overweight and toothless. Brian said that the Canadian government had put the First Nations folks on a beer ration of 12 beers per day and that we'd probably be asked to buy booze for someone who'd managed to burn through the day's allotment before dinnertime. At the far end of town, there was a restaurant and bar called the Snowshoe Inn. Inside, the pleather-padded metal dining chairs, Formica-topped tables, dark wood paneling, and dim lights transported us back to the 1980s, when the reason a middle-class family dined out was so the parents could sip cocktails in relative peace while the children played pinball and Pac-Man. As we ate our dinner of bison burgers, wings, and fries smothered in gravy, a steady stream of locals came in to buy their day's beer ration.

Across the street from the bar was the town's only motel. Judging by government license plates, we figured most of the clientele were forest and wildlife types. The bartender who served us our dinner and drinks told us the same women owned both the Snowshoe Inn and the motel. Brian left me in the bar to fend off a local who spoke to me in French, while he went across the street and asked about a place in town where we might pitch our tent. Ten minutes later, Brian returned and said the flat grassy spot at the top of the hill overlooking the public boat launch was available. "Apparently, that's where all the canoeists camp," he said.

"That's an old burial ground you're pitching that on," a local called out to us as we unrolled our tent on the space we were told we could take for the night. "You'll be sleeping on bones." He and his buddy chuckled before taking a long pull from a can of beer—the ground below them was littered with crushed red cans.

At around three o'clock that next morning, Brian was roused by barreling and revving of pickup trucks and all-terrain vehicles zooming past our tent. I have no memory of waking up or hearing them honking their horns or shooting gravel at our tent. A few hours later, I awoke and dressed in the tent. It was only day four, but the air inside our little sanctuary reeked of unwashed bodies, greasy hair, dirty socks, and dehydrated farts. After emerging from the tent, I headed down the bluff to collect our cooking supplies. There I discovered our canoe had been ransacked. The canoe itself was still tied up where we had left it, but someone had dumped the foodstuff from our bear canisters and threw them into the river. Fortunately, the two big canisters had floated back to shore, but the smaller one had not. They also dumped out our medical kit and the two large black duffel bags that contained most of our gear. The ground around the canoe and down to the shore looked as though a small bomb had exploded inside a sporting goods store.

I turned and stumbled up the bluff, feeling feeble, empty, and beaten. Brian was still in the tent, collecting himself for the day's paddle. After I told him what had happened, he bolted through the door of the tent and sprinted down the hill to the launch. As Brian ran through a mental checklist of supplies and took stock of what had been stolen or damaged, I collected the bear canisters from the shore, along with our waterlogged, formally shrink-wrapped cube of toilet paper. The thieves had taken the paleo bars and our pemmican. They also took Brian's handmade Hudson Bay axe, which wasn't cheap, though they left several other items that were equally as valuable. They also took the multi-purpose stove that would burn any fuel. "It was probably a handful of teenagers acting stupid after too many beers," I said, in a lame attempt to make Brian feel better. "I did worse when I was that age."

"I don't care who the fuck did this or why," Brian snapped back at me. He was right. This wasn't just some trip that was in jeopardy—Brian's reputation and livelihood were on the line. "The joys of being an adventure book writer," I said, again trying to reframe the situation. "This will make for a great chapter in the book."

Brian seemed unamused and uncomforted by my words. I'm sure he thought I didn't know what the hell I was talking about. None of this could possibly mean as much to me as it did to him. Because I didn't know what else to do, I picked up the garbage left by the thieves. After discarding it in a bear-proof dumpster near the top of the boat launch, I found my toothbrush and toothpaste and brushed my teeth. "It helps," I told Brian, with a mouthful of minty suds when he gave me a funny look. I spit and rinsed. "It's an old trick I learned while getting certified in college to fight forest fires. No matter how tired and dirty and deflated you are, stopping to brush your teeth always helps you feel better."

While Brian hiked back into town to report what had happened, I repacked what gear we had left and stood guard in the already blazing-hot morning sun. About an hour later, Brian returned with a couple shopping bags worth of replacement supplies he'd gathered from the only store in town. He handed me a Snickers bar. "Chocolate always helps, too," he said with a knowing smile.

In addition to the Royal Canadian Mounted Police—the RCMP, not "Mounties," I was warned—Brian had also called Doug Swallow, the gentleman he had rented the canoe from. Brian told me that Doug seemed genuinely wounded by what had happened to us and offered to hand-deliver another bear canister and a stove with fuel. "Doug says that in two-plus decades in business, something like this has never happened to any of his customers," Brian said while pulling out his toothbrush. "I guess we're the lucky ones."

When the officer arrived an hour or so later, she took our statements, commiserating with our distress as we described what had been taken and what had been destroyed. When Brian showed her the sopping-wet cube of now useless toilet paper, she reacted in a way I hadn't expected. "Dicks!" she shouted. "Am I right?" She was a brunette with a tight ponytail—"vaguely Italian," Brian thought—brusque yet cordial and compassionate. She told us she'd been up most of the night following up on break-ins all over the area. She tried to convince us that it wasn't anything personal, that we didn't do anything wrong. Merely a crime of opportunity is all. "Happens more than you'd think," she said.

— — —

The book Brian wrote about his journey down the Mackenzie River— *Disappointment River: Finding and Losing the Northwest Passage*—was published two years after I returned home from the Arctic. In April 2017, Brian sent me a polished draft of the chapter I was featured in; he said he wanted me to look for any factual errors and to let him know if he had written anything that didn't mesh with what I remembered.

"David Chrisinger is a big man, a former college football defensive tackle with a soft polite voice and a dense red beard," Brian began. "He grew up deer hunting with his grandfather, a game warden in central Wisconsin, a place I used to think of as prohibitively northern. I laugh at such thoughts now."[1] Two pages later, Brian commented on my size again: "Once at the lake . . . our top-heavy canoe wobbled as breeze-blown rollers came in off the open water. David and I had never paddled together, and we would never be heavier, I realized. So much food, plus David, the largest of my companions."[2] And again, two pages after that: "David and I decided to switch places. I had started the trip in the back, my traditional place as a guide, but we wanted to see if the canoe handled better with his greater weight in the rear," Brian writes.[3]

I read Brian's chapter about my portion of the journey in fits and starts between sessions of a writing seminar I was teaching at Columbia University in New York City. Before I had a chance to finish reading, Ashley called to see how my week of teaching was going. I told her that Brian had sent me a chapter to read and that he must have some complex about my size, considering that he felt the need to mention it in three separate passages in the span of a handful of pages. Ashley, a dietitian, had been trying to help me lose the weight I'd gained since taking off my football pads for the last time. As she did whenever I felt disparaged about my weight, she reminded me that, yes, I have a large body, but it's an athletic body. "Well, you can't tell that from what Brian wrote," I snapped back at her.

"Can you send it to me?" Ashley asked. "I'd love to read Brian's side of your trip together."

After I had finished teaching the last session of the day, I checked my phone and saw a text from Ashley. "Read the rest of the chapter," the message read. "It makes more sense why Brian had to mention how big you are once you get to the part about the storm."

— — —

I discovered Brian's first book, *The Long Walk*, at the Hudson Booksellers outside gate A7 at the Seattle-Tacoma International Airport. Before the flight attendant had finished her safety instructions, I stopped reading and slipped it back into my computer bag. It wasn't what I had expected. "The first thing you should know about me," it begins, "is that I'm Crazy. I haven't always been. Until that one day, the day I went Crazy, I was fine. Or I thought I was. Not anymore."[4] From there, it gets even more intense, even more confessional.

A few days later, unable to sleep, I picked it back up. As my wife drifted off to sleep next to me, my heartbeat sped up as I turned the pages. My first impression of the book had been totally off. This was not some spill-your-guts recounting of the horrors of war, nor was it the bland historical recounting I had grown accustomed to in graduate school. It was a transformation, a source of discoveries and recognitions. In it Brian exposes his bomb-damaged brain, not to drive the reader away, but to bring both himself and the reader closer to the truth. I felt stretched. For the next couple of days, Brian's book was where I lived. After having read through it on the first pass almost at a run, my excitement conquering my desire to slow down and savor, I started back at the beginning, reluctant to be separated from it. On the second pass, I held myself to the pace the book merited and even read some of it aloud, a chapter each night before bed.

"Listen to this," I said to Ashley, who was rocking our son in the dark-wood rocking chair near our bed. "My wife is alone in our full bed too," I began:

> Her husband, the father of her children, never came back from Iraq. When I deployed the first time she asked her grandmother for advice. Her grandfather served in Africa and Europe in World War II. Her grandmother would know what to do.
>
> "How do I live with him being gone? How do I help him when he comes home?" my wife asked.
>
> "He won't come home," her grandmother answered. "The war will kill him one way or the other. I hope for you that he dies while he is there. Otherwise the war will kill him at home. With you."[5]

"That's very powerful," my wife said in a whisper, trying not to disturb our son, who had just fallen asleep.

"That's damn near the exact same thing my grandmother told some friend at my grandfather's funeral," I said before returning to the book. I paused with Brian's book in my lap. "It's just," I said, "my grandfather was such a miserable bastard, just an embarrassing disappointment. My dad has never said a nice word about him."

I paused, searching for the right words. "He never fit the mold," I continued. "I don't know how to explain it. He wasn't like what you see in *Band of Brothers* or any of that Greatest Generation stuff the History Channel churns out." I looked down again at the book and read on: "I sleep alone," Brian writes, "with the Crazy. And its gray spidery fingers take the top of my head off to eat my brain and heart from the inside out every night as I stare at the ceiling in my solitary bed."[6] Is that what my grandfather felt, too?

Looking up at Ashley once more, I stopped. "Now I read this," I said, "and I don't know. Maybe my grandfather wasn't that abnormal or whatever, you know?"

"You should see if you can find his email somewhere," she said, standing up from the rocking chair. She placed our son in the pack-and-play next to our bed and climbed in under the tan comforter. She wrapped her left arm around my midsection, her head against my chest. "Tell him how much his book meant to you," she said without looking up at me. "I bet he'd like to know."

I clicked off the lamp next to our bed and placed Brian's book on the nightstand. Unable to sleep, I thought about how inconceivable it was that I could be in contact with him. He wasn't supposed to have fans who could interrupt his privacy. As I was reading and being borne aloft by *The Long Walk*, I never stopped to think that Brian was a real flesh-and-blood person, that he was literally *here*. For me, he was a book, a story that made so much of my life—and my family's history—come into sharp focus after years of blurriness. As far as I was concerned, Brian Castner was as fictional as Hemingway's Frederic Henry or Heller's John Yossarian. Why would he even need to talk to me? I had his book. What else was there to talk about?

— — —

Brian's goal for day four was to snake through a series of small islands to where the Mackenzie River widened into Mills Lake. According to the guidebook, it wasn't uncommon for canoeists to get stranded on Mills Lake for a day or two. The lake is so shallow that when the wind picks up just a little, whitecaps can whip up and make it impossible to keep going.

Much to our surprise and delight, the water in Mills Lake was flat and calm, not a whitecap to be seen. The sky was a brilliant blue, so blue in fact that could I have dipped my hand into it, my gloved fingers would have come back wet with paint. I'm not much of a churchgoer, but the landscape that day stirred something spiritual in me. To the north there no longer seemed to be any sort of horizon. There was only a majestic blue panorama of sky and water, a near-perfect mirror that reflected all that was beautiful and calming about this place. Instead of stopping for the day as Brian had originally planned, we skirted the southern shore without any trouble from wind or waves, feeling fortunate for the first time all week. From the back of the canoe, I steered us from point to point along the shore, careful not to get too far from land.

Brian's back was starting to bother him, he said, and his shoulders were stiff and sore from all the paddling. Each time he pinched his shoulder blades together or arched the small of his back, I could hear the pops and groans of his battered body. I was then suddenly aware of Brian's intense need for dedicated quiet, a quiet I don't think I've ever experienced with another human being. I became self-conscious of all the questions I had been asking him about writing and being an author and whatever else my curiosity suggested.

For the first time all week, I went nearly an hour in the canoe without saying a word. Before too long, the pent-up anxiety, now released, paired with general exhaustion, the rhythmic nature of my paddle stroke, and the sound of the canoe cutting through the water all resulted in a meditative calm that eventually ended with my head slumping forward and then suddenly jerking back. Not wanting to fall fast asleep and go over the side of the canoe, I did the only thing I thought would keep me awake: I talked. Because Brian had cut me off the last time I brought it up, I started with my trip to Okinawa, not caring if Brian was listening or not. Simply saying my thoughts out loud, I convinced myself, would help me make sense of them. If Brian added his two cents, that would simply be icing on the cake. I talked about what a strange place Okinawa was and how commercial and developed it had become. Brian said he was surprised I had brought Ashley with me. He said that he'd never thought to include his wife on a research or writing trip but that she would probably be overjoyed to be asked. "My wife's love language is quality time," I said, citing the insights of *The Five Love Languages*. "Mine, too," Brian said in a soft, contemplative tone.

As though I had rehearsed what I would say if finally given the opportunity to speak, I found a nice, unstrained rhythm of play-by-play recounting. The highlight of the trip, I told Brian, was the second-to-last day, when Ashley and I met up with American expat Jack Letscher, who worked in his spare time as a battlefield historian. The morning we met him at our hotel, he handed me a short stack of photocopied topographical maps that were divided into neat grids and further divided into smaller squares. Certain squares on each page were highlighted, and he explained that he'd taken records of my grandfather's company and traced the routes the men had taken and the places they had fought onto the copies of the battlefield maps I now held in my hand. For the next eight hours or so, he took us along the same routes in the same order that my grandfather's company had once traversed. Brian listened without interrupting or asking questions. Then I told him about my father and what a difficult relationship I had with him and how my journey to uncover the truth and write a book about his father was a sort of pilgrimage I had created for myself to bring my father some peace.

"Like *Field of Dreams*," Brian said.

"Yeah, I guess. I never thought about it like that," I said, thinking of the 1989 movie starring Kevin Costner in which a farmer in Iowa builds a baseball field at the edge of his cornfield to ease his long-dead father's pain.

"You know, though," Brian continued, "it wasn't his father who needed peace. It was Costner."

"That's true."

"Do you want some advice?" he asked, as if he had finally realized that is all I wanted all along. "You need to figure out what peace you were looking for," he said.

"Okay," I said and thought for a moment. "I guess I don't know exactly."

"Figure that out, and you'll have yourself a book," Brian said with a candid authority for which I held a respectful appreciation.

Finally I was getting what I wanted, what I had been waiting for. Yes, I'd sat on a plane for two days and flew 4,000 miles from home to the Arctic to escape some of the drama of my life and recharge whatever batteries I had left, and, yes, I'd thought I would be able to help a hero of mine in a time of need, but really what I was looking for was his advice.

I thought for a moment about what peace I was looking for. Then Brian interjected another thought: "Unless you know what you, as the writer and as one of the main characters, actually wants, all you're going to have is a bunch of pages where a bunch of stuff happens, but none of it matters because that's all it is—just a bunch of stuff a reader has no particular reason to care about."

Then he asked me something I hadn't anticipated: "Why do you want to be a full-time author anyway? You've put out a couple books already. Clearly your job isn't so demanding that you don't have the time or energy to work on stuff that's important to you. Plus, I bet your pay and benefits are good."

"And I have a pension," I added.

"Shit," he said, adjusting the brim of his hat between paddle strokes. "If I had flexibility and time and a salary and benefits and a pension, I wouldn't be out here for 40 days—away from my wife and kids—trying to scrape up enough material to fill a book no one's going to remember after I'm dead and gone."

"How can you say that?" I asked incredulously.

"Tell me this," he continued, ignoring my question. "Why do you *really* want to write this book? You writing a book isn't going to bring your father any peace; you could just tell him what you found if that's all you want."

"I suppose it's like what Twain said. If you want to be remembered, you either have to write a book or do something worth writing a book about."

"Unless your last name is Washington or Lincoln," Brian replied, "no one's going to remember you a generation or two after you're gone. No book is going to change that." He continued, "This life ain't all it's cracked up to be. Believe me."

"Well," I said, "if you think what I have is so great, you should apply. We're trying to fill like six of my positions."

Later that day, over peanut butter and honey wraps and fruit, Brian confided in me that his first book had sold for big money. He said that he was almost embarrassed by how much and that he was never going to make back the advance he received. His second book, however, was rejected by the publisher who had bought his first one. The editor he worked with on *The Long Walk* told Brian that maybe he had only one book in him. "He said that Michael Herr only wrote one book too—*Dispatches*—and that I shouldn't be too hard on myself," Brian said.

"Man, what a dick," I replied with a mouth full of food.

"Yeah, but then that same guy is my editor for this book, so . . ."

To sell his second book, Brian had completely restructured it. Twice. I started to wonder whether Brian's experience with his second book was making him a better teacher of writing and whether he was practicing his chops on me. I've learned through my dealings in the writing world that good writers aren't always good teachers. Often the opposite is true because most people are better at teaching something they've learned through experience, through trial and error, than they are at teaching something they somehow innately know. When someone like Brian knows in his bones how to tell an intimate, vulnerable personal story, it can be easy to assume anyone can do the same. The person just has to want it badly enough. *Write a better book. It's that simple.* The cognitive unconscious of natural writers has a knack for offering up beautiful prose in story form, affording them the rare ability to write automatically—so automatically that it's easy to believe that's the nature of writing itself, rather than simply their nature.

Natural storytellers aren't normally equipped with the tools to deconstruct what they've done or to pinpoint what it is that a reader will respond to—not until they get knocked on their ass and are forced to figure it out for themselves. Their debut books are beautiful and haunting and stick with you for days after you finish them. But because they can't put their finger on what made it so captivating, their second books can oftentimes fall flat in comparison.

The next available campsite was another 8 or 10 miles down the river, on the northern shore. There we found a perfect camping spot with plenty of breeze and very few mosquitos. The shore was sandy and full of seashells. Seagulls chatted in the background. The scenery reminded me of pictures I have seen of Alaska, the wide and long valleys that were carved out by glaciers and are now dotted with rocks and low bushes, a land teeming with wildlife. To the north of us, dark purple clouds fluffed by. An occasional lighting strike diverted my attention from the camp chores. They were close enough to see but far enough away not to worry about. To the west, the sun kissed the tops of the distant trees. Brian sat on a flat rock with his legs crossed, jotting notes in his journal as I pitched the tent and filled up our water bottles.

Why Does It Matter How You Describe Your Characters?

The day after our craft talk, Brian and I were making good time in a section of the river that had a nice steady current. We had made up more than enough miles by that point in the trip, so when we saw the black monster clouds ballooning in great rolls and zooming in from the west, Brian didn't hesitate to call it a day.

As a black sky descended upon us, Brian and I quickly set the tent up on a sandy stretch of beach along the northern shore of the river, with the front end of it pointing directly into the wind. We figured that because the tent was so aerodynamic, it stood a better chance of surviving the storm if it faced into the wind. Just as I staked in the rear grommets, the air around me felt like the temperature had dropped 20 or 30 degrees. We both crawled inside the tent and braced ourselves.

Within 10 minutes or so, the storm was pounding and rattling the walls of the tent. Rain fell in sheets and columns; lightning shattered the air into quaking pieces. To stave off my anxiety, I jotted notes in my journal. The coolness of the floor on my back was a welcome reprieve from the intensity of the Arctic sun. To be honest, I was happy to be out of the canoe and away from the mind-numbing, monochromatic sameness the river had become.

The stakes holding in the front vestibule ripped out first; the thin spikes of metal banged against the top and sides of the tent. The dark, noisy slamming of the wind and rain intensified.

"It's okay," I said, trying to comfort myself as much as I was trying to reassure Brian. "It's not like it's going to blow away with us in it."

A second or two later, the rear stakes ripped up as well, and half the tent collapsed with us inside. I crawled out the front entryway and right into the teeth of the storm. The water was as black as the sky, and white-capped waves were crashing against the shore, gaining ground.

It was too windy, and the shore too soft, to stake the tent back down. I cursed into the wind as Brian retreated through the back door of the tent. Like me, he was standing bare-chested in his underwear, his hair plastered down onto his forehead. He pointed to the tree line behind us and yelled over the wind that maybe it was calmer up there. Brian stayed put to hold onto the tent and keep it from being blown into the river's oblivion as I darted up the shallow embankment and charged into the woods.

On the other side of a recently downed poplar, I found a small opening I thought was big enough for the tent. Determined to make it work, I pulled a clump of small plants from the earth with my bare hands, unsure of how firmly rooted they would be. Recoiling with sharp pain, I looked down at my calloused hands and saw dozens of black thorns stuck into the flesh of my palms and in the underside of my fingers. The small clearing was clogged with what I later learned were prickly primrose plants. With the rumbling clouds booming at my back, I pulled the biggest plants out completely and stomped down the smaller ones. My hands swelled and bled.

After clearing out as many plants as I could, I ran back down to Brian and told him about the spot. He nodded and collapsed the tent like an accordion with our sleeping bags and mats still inside. As if he were back in a war zone barking out orders, he told me to help him lift the tent off the ground and hike it up the shore like a pair of hobos carrying their only possessions wrapped in a giant handkerchief. Once we reached the tree line, the tent snagged on a branch poking up from the deadfall. Brian shook his head and yelled for us to stop so that we didn't accidently rip the tent beyond repair.

Leaving me with the tent accordion, Brian dashed back to the shore to grab the backpack in which we stored our wallets, passports, and electronics. After dumping the backpack at my feet, he returned to the shore to grab more gear and found that the worst of the front had passed and that the wind was merely howling. Instead of camping in the trees that night, he decided we were going to stake the tent back down on the shore. And if we had to stand there holding it until the front passed, that's what we were going to do.

With the tent back on the shore and stretched out to its full footprint, we used the extra stakes Brian packed to tie down the support lanyards, which is what climbers must do on Everest to keep a tent like Brian's from blowing away. Once all the stakes were in, I hiked up and down the shore, grabbing stones the size of basketballs to place over each of the stakes. I didn't know whether the extra weight would make any difference, but it felt good to be doing something, anything that seemed even remotely productive.

Here's how Brian described what happened next: "When it looked like the tent was out of danger, David single-handedly dragged the half-loaded canoe up the beach until it was level with the shelter. With much of our gear, not to mention all our food, still inside, it weighed at least five hundred pounds."[7]

Would you have believed what Brian wrote if you didn't already know that I was a large man, a former college football player? What initially struck me as a needlessly repetitive description of my size turned out to serve a specific purpose in Brian's story. In his description of me, he was establishing the readers' expectations so that my actions during an important and dramatic moment in the story would be surprising yet inevitable.

—— —— ——

Several days later, I looked out the window of the Mackenzie Rest Inn and saw Brian and Jeremy, Brian's next paddling companion, float by along the southern shore of the river. Brian was back in his rightful place—in the rear of the canoe—paddling with intensity. Jeremy was adjusting his bug net over his long brown beard, his canoe paddle laid across his lap. I felt a longing mixed with a sense of desperation, like I was experiencing withdrawal for something my body thought it badly needed.

My knees felt weak, and a lump started to form in my throat as I thought back to the last thing Brian had said to me before we parted. Jeremy had just arrived, and Brian was anxious to get packed and back on the water. He hugged me tight around the shoulders and held on for a moment longer than I thought he would. "I'll text you," he said. "Love you, brother."

Feeling much better after having showered, brushed my teeth, and washed my clothes in the tub, I logged on to Wi-Fi to delete most of the emails and messages I'd missed by being off the grid for the previous 10 days. My phone sprung to life, vibrating with each newly loaded message and notification. It took a few minutes before it finished. The grand total: 62 Gmails, 55 Facebook notifications, 5 Facebook messages, and 109 work emails. With the snap of the digital finger, I was no longer on a wilderness adventure; I was back to real life.

I checked my work emails first. It looked like I didn't miss too much. Dozens of messages that didn't require any action from me. All except for one—an email from by supervisor. I forgot to validate my time card. When I opened my Facebook messages, I found one from my renter saying he had finally moved all his stuff out of the house and was sorry he'd been such an asshole about everything. I couldn't respond. I needed to think about what I was going to say to him.

The last of the Facebook messages was from my father. It was time-stamped the same day that Brian and I crossed Beaver Lake. The day he had helped me figure out how to solve the problem with my book. My father wrote that he'd been trying to call for two days about my son's soccer schedule but that I hadn't bothered to call him back. I know I sent him a message about my trip, or did I tell him over the phone? I must have told him I'd be out of touch for a couple of weeks. Confused, I read the next message he sent: "You don't want me in your life, fine, your choice," it began. "Circle of life, my father didn't want me either, now you don't want me. No idea what the problem is, at this point don't care. So long, adios."

———   ———   ———

I wish I could remember the chain of thoughts that led me to this, but for whatever reason, while I was lying in bed at the Mackenzie Rest Inn, I started thinking about "fatal flaws" in literature. All those fundamental misbeliefs that keep main characters in stories from living the life they want. Mr. Santy, my freshman English teacher in high school, taught me how to spot fatal flaws in the fall of 2001. Ground zero was still smoldering in lower Manhattan, and while first responders and good Samaritans continued to dig through the rubble, I sat uncomfortably in a plastic desk chair, more than a thousand miles away, reading E. B. White's *Charlotte's Web*. The main character was a pig named Wilbur, and during a discussion in class, I realized that Wilbur's fatal flaw was that he so feared death and loss that he was unable to enjoy what life he had left. I remember thinking that such flaws didn't exist for real people, at least not in the way it worked in books. I didn't think it was possible to boil down a real person into a single hamstringing misbelief. Or maybe I just never wanted to acknowledge in myself such dark, barely perceivable spider-web cracks that spread across a life.

After spending 10 days in a canoe with Brian, I started thinking that maybe life was more like literature than I had cared to admit. Maybe what I perceived as reality was nothing more than the stories I told myself, and maybe fatal flaws really did exist, after all.

What was my grandfather's fatal flaw? There was something about his inability to confide fully in another person, his penchant for silence and secrecy, violence and rage. There were other flaws, too.

And what about my father? He struggled most of his life to overcome some deep sense of shame, which manifested itself in self-deprecation, feelings of worthlessness, and panic.

What about me?

A couple of months after I returned from Canada, on a cool fall morning, I asked my wife what she thought my fatal flaw was. After the words left my mouth, she looked up at me with her beautiful hazel eyes, her steaming cup of coffee poised at her lips. Her expression was wry. "That's easy," she said. "You think you're responsible for other people's happiness. You think you can protect people from the bad stuff in their lives and that will make them happy."

When I told my mother, a few days later, what Ashley had said and how I thought she was right, my mother told me over the phone about the time, years and years ago, when she ran into my kindergarten teacher at the grocery store. My teacher was a little concerned about me, she told my mother, because earlier that week, when it was my turn to pass out the straws at morning milk break, I broke into tears after running out of straws. Through my inconsolable sobs, I told her that I had run out of straws, that it was all my fault, and that I had let my friends down.

Then there was my undying need for my father's validation, which she illustrated using a handful of stories I had only vague memories of. This was not something we had ever discussed before, and she wasn't sure why she never talked to me about it. "It's so easy, isn't it," she said, "to see the flaws in each other right away? It's much harder to see our own."

— — —

The closest I've ever come to combat was the day I sat in the Marine recruiter's office almost three years after the Twin Towers fell. It was late July, and I was itching to leave the small town I grew up in and do something that felt important. There was a war on, and in my family, when our nation was at war, the men had always done their part.

On September 11, 2001, I watched United Airlines Flight 175 slam into the south face of the South Tower on live television. I was sitting in homeroom before first period, watching *Good Morning America* on a bulky television suspended from the ceiling in a corner of the classroom. I remember Charles Gibson and Diane Sawyer announcing that a plane had crashed into the World Trade Center. My teacher flipped the channel to CNN. The commentators there were speculating about what could have caused such a tragic accident. Then it happened. The second plane hit.

I sat there in stunned disbelief with the rest of my class for what seemed like forever. The bell rang, and life pressed us to move on. We stumbled into the hallway and made our way to our next classes. The halls buzzed with talk of what had happened. One student in my grade said his dad was in New York on business and was supposed to have had a meeting at the World Trade Center. That turned out to be bullshit. None of us knew anyone in New York City, or DC for that matter. We were as insulated in our small town as anyone could have been.

Over the next couple of days, we learned that Osama bin Laden was behind the attacks. We watched President George W. Bush shout through a megaphone to a mass of first responders that the people who knocked down the Twin Towers would be hearing from us soon. I watched Bruce Springsteen sing about his "city of ruins" during the

Concert for New York City. Our school staged our own fundraiser. The glee club sang Lee Greenwood's "Proud to Be an American," and the National Honor Society sold medical wristbands for a dollar with the name of someone who had been killed on 9/11 written in black marker. I wore the wristband I bought for weeks. I wish I still had it. I can't remember the name.

Then life went on. I played football and went to homecoming with a girl named Val, wrote term papers and studied for Spanish 2 exams. Basketball season started in November. Baseball in the spring. As a nation, we were at war, but it didn't feel like it to me. I didn't know anyone who was serving, let alone someone who had been deployed overseas. I remember after Christmas hearing that we had won the war in Afghanistan.

Soon enough, our television sets began blaring about Iraq. It was in the news for months, but I don't remember talking about it at school or around the dinner table. The clearest thing I do remember was how confident the president seemed, like he knew something vital about Iraq's weapons of mass destruction and Saddam Hussein's intentions to use them that he couldn't tell us. Behind all their public certainty, the Bush administration knew that the evidence they were using to support many of their claims was limited at best, and there were many discrepancies between what the president was saying publicly and the intelligence information that was available at the time. The administration presented its claims as facts anyway. We know now, of course, that this confidence was masking the known unknown. But back then, to my teenage brain, the world was black and white, right and wrong, good and evil, and the president's logic appealed to that worldview. I was just barely old enough to drive, and my prefrontal cortex wasn't fully developed yet; I couldn't process consequences. That was my excuse. I don't know what the president's was.

On the day American forces invaded Iraq, in March 2003, I was in Madison, Wisconsin, with my father and brother. Every year around that time, we would drive three and a half hours south to Madison to attend the annual state tournament for high school boys basketball. We watched the "shock and awe" footage from the invasion on the news in our hotel room. We would be fighting in the streets of Iraq, the president said, so that we would not have to fight in our own streets those terrorists who wished us harm. "I've heard that before," my father said to himself, after taking a long pull from his can of Diet Mountain Dew. Two nights before, on Saint Patrick's Day, President Bush had addressed the nation. He said the United Nations Security Council had not lived up to its responsibilities. "So we will rise to ours," he said. "We are now acting because the risks of inaction would be far greater."

The University of Wisconsin in Madison has a history of protests against ill-advised wars, and the day after the invasion began, a mass of protesters assembled outside the state capitol to continue the tradition. In between basketball games, my dad decided to walk us down there to watch what was happening. For such a historic moment, it left me wanting. From the outside, the protest seemed disorganized. The protestors carried colorful and creatively worded signs, but the protest itself was characterized largely by agitprop, inchoate rage, and lefty piety. They had no story to combat the president's version of things, and that made it hard to take them seriously. They looked like hippies out of a history textbook and seemed almost deluded by their ideals of peace. Didn't they know there were people out there who wanted to kill us?

Years after the invasion, my father told me he had never supported it. I don't dispute that, but I also don't remember him saying as much. The fight of my generation was about to begin, and honestly, it didn't matter to me if the president was exactly right—or if my father supported it. Saddam was bad. We were good. When my friends started to enlist, they did so at a more innocent and optimistic point in the war. Military service carried no stigma where we lived. The torture photos from Abu Ghraib hadn't yet leaked. The Haditha massacre hadn't yet occurred. We hadn't yet completely fumbled the occupation. Hundreds of thousands of Iraqis had not yet been killed.

"Why do you want to be a Marine?" the recruiter asked that hot July afternoon in the summer of 2004. "I want to make a difference," I told him. "And I want to be the best." I thought that was what he wanted to hear. The truth was that I wanted my father to be proud of me. He told me once that not getting to serve in Vietnam was one of the greatest regrets of his life.

The recruiter leaned back in his metal chair, behind his gunmetal tanker desk. He stared at me. "You think you have what it takes?" he asked. He was sizing me up, trying to figure out which sales pitch I would respond to best. A choose-your-own-adventure way of convincing young men and women to serve. I didn't need any convincing, though. I was already sold.

A week after my visit to the recruiter, I broke the news to my father while we were shooting hoops at the YMCA. He had just come off the day shift at the paper mill, and it was his day off. I knew he'd be his most relaxed—and most receptive—on a day like that. Basketball had always calmed his nerves. When he played, he entered some kind of flow state that lowered his blood pressure and reminded him of better times. When he was in high school, my father was a lights-out shooter, and even in his older age, despite all the troubles he had with his knees and back, he could still drain it from anywhere on the court. I wanted to enlist as soon as I was able, so after my father had sunk a few three-pointers from the corner, I blurted out that I wanted to join the Marines and that I wanted to go to Iraq.

I passed back the ball. He caught it and held it like a football. "Have you talked to your mother?" he asked. "Not yet," I said. "I was hoping you could help me make the case to her."

My father looked down at his watch. "Hey, we better get you to work. You're going to be late," he said. I could tell he wasn't ready to hear what I had said. He dropped me off at the home improvement store, where I stocked shelves, swept floors, and helped unappreciative contractors load 50-pound bags of cement into rusted work trucks.

An hour before closing time, my father returned to the store and found me stocking aluminum elbows for downspouts. He looked like he was on a mission—eyes focused on me, arms swinging at his side. He waved his hand as I opened my mouth to ask what he was doing there.

"Just let me say what I need to before you respond," he said. "First, I get why you'd want to join. I really do. I've been there myself. The thing is . . ." He stopped to collect his thoughts. "The thing is that I just don't feel good about Iraq."

My father's no dove. He believes strongly that if America's national security interests dictate that we send our troops into harm's way, we should do so, but he knows firsthand how war damages the minds and bodies of the troops that fight them.

"I know you think the Marines is going to make a man out of you," he continued, "but that's bullshit, and I need you to know that. Don't let anyone convince you otherwise." He paused again. "Do you know what makes a man?" he asked. "A man busts his ass to give his children a better life. I've been at the mill 20 years now, and all that time, the only thing that's kept me going is the thought that someday I'll be able to send you and your brother to college. Don't take that from me. Not like this."

I didn't know what to say. I couldn't argue with him. Part of me was relieved by how much he suddenly seemed to care for me. It was an unfamiliar feeling.

"Do you know what Marines do?" he asked after another pause. I thought it was a rhetorical question, so I said nothing. "They kill people. You know that, right?" He paused again, letting the words seep in. It was not something that had crossed my mind. "Are you ready to kill somebody? Is that what you want to do? Do you want to live with that?" Another long pause.

"This war is going to get messy; it's much more complicated than the news lets on, and it doesn't look like there's any end in sight," he continued. "And quite frankly, I don't want to see you get your ass shot off for people who don't seem to want our help. I don't want you to end up like your grandfather, either."

References

1. Brian Castner, *Disappointment River: Finding and Losing the Northwest Passage* (New York: Doubleday, 2018), 139.

2. Castner, *Disappointment River*, 141.

3. Castner, *Disappointment River*, 143.

4. Brian Castner, *The Long Walk: A Story of War and the Life That Follows* (New York: Anchor Books, 2012), 1.

5. Castner, *Long Walk*, 89–90.

6. Castner, *Long Walk*, 91.

7. Castner, *Disappointment River*, 155.

PART II The Structure

Incorporating the Five Essentials of Storytelling

I THREW Brett a going-away party at my mother's house the night before he left for boot camp. It was the summer of 2005, about a month after we graduated from high school. My mother was out of town visiting her old college friends. While most of our friends who showed up sat in the living room drinking cheap beer or on the rusted deck chairs behind the house smoking menthol cigarettes, Brett and I crawled out my second-floor bedroom window onto the roof of the front porch. The night was cool and dry, and for a couple hours we sat there, sipping cans of Miller Lite he had taken from his old man.

My mother's house was sided in dark-stained wood and shielded from a busy intersection by a stand of dense trees and shrubs. The street light that normally illuminated the four-way stop had burned out; Brett and I watched car after car approach the intersection, miss the stop sign, slam on the breaks at the last minute, and skid through to the other side. We chuckled every time. Parked on the side of the street in front of my mother's house was a light royal blue 1984 Buick Century with a sagging headliner and a crumpled front passenger door. My father had bought it for me the year I turned 16. The second time I pulled it out of the garage I crashed into a split-rail fence during a snowstorm. For two years I drove that thing—until one day when I couldn't get it to start. By then my father was looking for a new vehicle for himself, so he offered to sell me his 1997 Chevy 1500 if I could find a buyer for the Buick. Brett took one look at it, knew he could get it running, and paid cash. He drove it all winter of our senior year and planned to flip it before he left for San Diego.

That night on the roof, the asphalt shingles abrasive under our ass cheeks, I didn't really know what to talk about with Brett. I asked him how the car was running. "Piece of shit," he said with a sly grin before taking a sip from his can. If he was nervous about leaving the next morning, I couldn't tell. If he asked me about how I was feeling about the next stage in my life, I don't remember. Mostly we just sat and drank.

Brett told me once that he could still remember Whitney's face when he told her he had enlisted. They were leaning up against Brett's car in the parking lot of Hardee's, on the east side of town. He just blurted it out. There had been no discussion. No consultation. Whitney felt hurt and dismayed. She thought their relationship meant more to Brett than it seemed to that day. She was also scared. Not about him being gone. It was more that he might not ever return or that he might not return the same man she loved.

When Brett told the recruiter he wanted to become a police officer after he got out, the recruiter told him he should serve as a presidential guard. Brett's plans changed during boot camp after he made friends with a few Marines who were on their way to becoming members of the Fleet Antiterrorism Security Team, FAST for short—though Brett told me that FAST really stood for "Fake Ass SEAL Team." The promise of travel and adventure that came with FAST sounded like a good deal to him. "The problem," Brett explained after he left the service, "is that no one considers FAST guys to be 'real Marines.' We're not in the shit in Iraq and Afghanistan."

That all changed one night in 2007. Brett and his FAST buddies were getting drunk in the barracks at Virginia Beach. An officer came into Brett's room and said he was looking for combat replacements who wanted to go to Iraq. Brett thought about it. No one in the room made a sound. He wouldn't be doing what he had been trained to do in FAST, but at least he could say he had been there—that he'd actually done something. That was all the convincing he needed. Brett raised his hand. He was the only one. "I know it's dumb, but looking back I was so proud of myself," Brett told me. "I showed I had the biggest balls in the room."

The Five Essentials of Storytelling

Oftentimes I'll start writing a story—or what I think might make a good story—only to run out of steam before I bother finishing. Sometimes I stop because I lose interest in the subject or because I don't think what I have to say is all that important, even though I know in the back of my mind that isn't true. Other times I stop because I can't figure out how to end the story or because the ending hasn't happened yet.

Because traumatic experiences are frequently unresolvable or difficult to make sense of, the stories we tell about them lack a resolution as well. I'm reminded, for example, of a story relayed to Michael Herr, a war correspondent who spent a year in Vietnam and later wrote a book titled *Dispatches* about his experiences there. Shortly after landing in country in 1967, Herr writes, he met a LURP who was on his third tour of duty. LURP is an Army acronym that stands for "long-range reconnaissance patrol," and in Vietnam, LURPs spent days and sometimes weeks at a time observing the enemy in the darkest reaches of the jungle.

"Patrol went up the mountain," the LURP said to Herr. "One man came back. He died before he could tell us what happened." Herr writes that he waited for the LURP to tell him the rest but soon realized that "it seemed not to be that kind of story."[1] When he asked what had happened next, the LURP eyed Herr with a look of pity. In that moment, Herr knew he had revealed to the grizzled veteran just how little he understood about Vietnam. Herr had arrived there believing that language and stories could bring form to the inscrutable and the inconclusive. He was wrong.

Later in the book, Herr circles back to this story and writes that it took him a full year in Vietnam to understand what the LURP had tried to convey to him that day. While Herr does not explain what he learned to his readers, one expert on American literature of the Vietnam War noted that the LURP's three-sentence narrative "has been used to illustrate the essence of the violent wartime experiences that can be related only in cryptic and elusive language." The LURP's story seems, in turn, "to sum up in a miniature the uncertainty, sudden death, and frustration of the war as it was experienced by so many. That, and not 'what happened next,' is the tale's 'meaning' in the context of *Dispatches*, and Herr could not fully grasp it until he'd escaped the misconception of combat operations as mostly under control and easily comprehensible."[2] *Dispatches* in general, and this story in particular, are devoid of resolution. They are parables. And one does not explain parables.

People who tell stories like the one Herr details in *Dispatches* generally receive negative responses from their audiences, according to Kate McLean, a professor of psychology at Western Washington University. "The redemptive story is really valued in America," McLean told Julie Beck for a 2015 article in the *Atlantic*, "because for a lot of people it's a great way to tell stories, but for people who just can't do that, who can't redeem their traumas for whatever reason, they're sort of in a double bind. They both have this crappy story that's hanging on, but they also can't tell it and get acceptance or validation from people."[3]

Jonathan Adler is a professor of psychology at Olin College of Engineering. His research may give us a clue as to what kind of story to tell when there isn't much redemption to be had. Through his research, Adler has noticed two themes in people's stories that tend to correlate with better personal well-being: (1) agency, a feeling that you are in control of your life, and (2) communion, a feeling that you have good relationships in your life.

When I begin to sense that a story I'm writing isn't making progress toward resolution, I find it helps to use a formula, especially if I am passionate about the piece and the only thing stopping me from finishing is the realization that reality—and what it takes to capture reality on the page—is unforgivingly complex. For centuries storytellers have used all manner of formulas, although one stands out above the rest: the dramatic arc.

Jane Alison is a professor of creative writing at the University of Virginia, and in March 2019 she published an essay in the *Paris Review* that briefly lays out the history of the dramatic arc. "Twenty-five hundred years ago," she writes, "Aristotle dissected tragedies such as Sophocles' *Oedipus the King* to find their common features, as he might dissect snakes to see if their spines were alike. He found that powerful dramas shared certain elements, including a particular path."[4] In the *Poetics*, Aristotle described what his dissections revealed: "A tragedy is an imitation of an action that is complete in itself [with a] beginning, middle, and end. . . . Every tragedy is in part Complication and in part Dénouement; the incidents before the opening scene, and often certain also of those within the play, forming the Complication; and the rest the Dénouement. By Complication I mean all from the beginning of the story to the point just before the change in the hero's fortunes; by Dénouement, all from the beginning of the change to the end."[5] Put simply, in dramatic stories a situation arises—either by cause or coincidence—tension builds and then reaches a peak, some action is taken, and then there is dénouement, a French word meaning "to untie the knot."

The dramatic arc—with its inciting event, progressive complications, crisis, climax, and resolution—is by no means the only way to structure a story. I have found in my classes and in my own writing, however, that if the goal is to tell personal stories of trauma, survival, and transformation that create connection and understanding, the five components of the dramatic arc—what I call the Five Essentials of Storytelling—are perfectly suited to the task. Unless writers employ the Five Essentials, they run the risk of presenting a story that may confuse, unsettle, or bore most readers.

As writers, we are competing with Netflix, smartphones, and a dozen other distractions that pull at our readers' attention. If the Five Essentials of Storytelling I lay out in this chapter seem too restrictive, please keep in mind that if your story either fails to meet your readers' unconscious expectations—or if you include information that doesn't fit into one of the Five Essentials—more often than not your story will not engage them. Your readers will feel as though they've been catapulted unceremoniously back into their own realities. I've found this to be true regardless of how beautifully the prose is written.

Once you have mastered the Five Essentials of Storytelling, you should feel emboldened to experiment with other shapes. My mother taught art for nearly three decades, and one lesson she taught me when I was one of her students that has stuck with me is this: once you've learned the rules of art, you are then free to break them at will. In the section of storytelling exercises, there is a worksheet for the Five Essentials of Storytelling.

The First Essential of Storytelling: The Inciting Event

The first essential of storytelling is the *inciting event*. The sole purpose of the inciting event is to knock the main character (you) out of their routine or upset the balance of their life in some way. An inciting event can occur in two ways: (1) either it occurs as the result of a choice that you or another character makes, or (2) it's a coincidence—that is, something unexpected, random, or accidental happens. In other words, *something* spurs you to act and begin your transformation. It can sometimes help to think about your object of desire and make your inciting event the moment you decided that's what you wanted.

In this chapter's story about Brett, I chose to throw a going-away party for him before he left for boot camp. Although I don't think I articulated it this way at the time, I was losing a friend—or at least a version of a friend. Part of me had to have known that Brett would be a different person the next time I saw him. How could he not be? I also knew that eventually he would be deployed and put in harm's way. And I knew that, in the summer of 2005, it seemed like the American death toll in Iraq would never level off. I was scared for him, and I felt uncomfortably out of sync for weeks after he left. Even after I settled into my own routine at college, I had to look at my reality in a new way. I had to adjust to the discomfort I felt about Brett living the current events I would be studying in a cavernous lecture hall.

There are two primary approaches to organization you can try when writing a personal narrative that I've found work well. The first is a straightforward chronology. I call this the "Keep it simple, Silly" way of writing memoir. That's what I used in this story about Brett. Before you twist yourself into knots coming up with a clever and unique way of telling your story, ask yourself whether it makes more sense simply to start at the beginning—the time when you started wanting your object of desire.

This sort of beginning usually includes a backstory or some exposition before the real action of the story begins that shows the reader what life looked like for you before the crisis, climax, and personal transformation (i.e., resolution) occurs (not to worry, we'll get to all that). Exposition is a fancy word for facts. It's the information you provide that helps the reader understand the setting, biography, and description of you and your characters—all the stuff your reader needs to know to follow and make sense of the events in your story.

I usually suggest that writers begin with a story that covers a relatively short period of time (say one to five years). There's not as much ground to cover between the chronological beginning and the crisis. If, on the other hand, your story covers more than five years of your life, a straightforward chronology may not work as well because there's much more ground to cover before your reader ever gets to the meat of the story. Keep in mind, though, that the more time you dedicate to providing background information and building tension, the more time you also give your reader to lose interest and see what's new on Netflix.

The trick to this approach is to make sure you start with a moment that is immediately gripping and dramatic. Then, during the rest of the setup, it's important to weave in multiple strands of meaning and nuance that will help the reader appreciate the beginning in a new way later in the story. Remember that the most important thing your beginning needs to do is get to the emotional core of your story as quickly as possible. What is at the heart of what you need to say? Whatever it is, start there.

The second approach you could take is often called in medias res, which means to start in the middle. (The Latin phrase in medias res translates as "in the midst of things"). If the chronological beginning to your story isn't the most interesting part, you may decide to start in the middle. Starting in the middle, where the action begins—or soon after it ends—can help hook your readers and make them feel more invested in you as a character. After you've got them hooked, you can then provide exposition that gives them a sense of what you were like before the crisis moment and perhaps why you behaved the way you did. Your reader is more likely to read through this information because you have provided a glimpse of the action that lies ahead for them. They will want to see how the crisis is eventually resolved.

Whichever approach to shaping your story you decide to take, the reader will feel more invested in your story when you include in the inciting event what I call grounding information. When did your story take place? Where did it take place? Who else besides you were involved? What is the situation? This story about Brett, for instance, begins in the summer of 2005, after Brett and I graduated from high school. We grew up in northern Wisconsin. Now Brett was headed to boot camp in California, and I was headed to college at a small state school 90 minutes south of where we grew up. Brett and I are the two main characters, although his girlfriend, Whitney, plays a supporting role. The goal in beginning your story is to situate readers in a specific time and place so that they can understand the landscape—both physical and emotional—as quickly as possible. Having a strong beginning to anchor your story can help bring your story's overall shape into focus and help you feel in control of the narrative as it develops.

— — —

The enormity of the grief Brett brought back with him from Afghanistan and his overpowering sense of loss were simply too much for him to process at first, let alone share with Whitney. Instead, he acted angry, abrupt. He didn't understand why, and he felt there wasn't much he could do about it. He was living in a strange world where the rules and conditions were quite different from those he had grown accustomed to in the Marine Corps. Once the anger subsided, depression would set in. Even though he had a job and was going to school, he felt out of place and unimportant. His own perception that he was somehow insignificant, coupled with the trauma he had experienced, was what hurt the most—and what caused the most despair.

For months after Brett first got home, Whitney felt like it was her responsibility not only to understand what Brett had been through but also to make things easier on him. In a sense, she felt that she needed to grieve for Brett. She eventually realized that while she could love and support him, Brett had to want to help himself. He needed to make changes and find a new sense of purpose. "It was really, really difficult," Whitney told me, "because there were times when I didn't want to be by his side, when he treated me poorly, when I actually packed my bags and drove three hours to my parents' house in the middle of the night because I couldn't stand to be around him for another second."

After months of emailing back and forth with Brett while I was still living in DC, I compiled all of the stories he had sent me into a semi-coherent Word document and organized them into a timeline from when he left home to when he and I reconnected online. What had once been fragments of thought became a sort of mosaic. I wish I could have seen his face when he opened the document; he had written more for me than he had ever written about anything else. He had told his stories, wrapped his arms around them in a way that made them coherent and meaningful.

The first time a story I wrote about Brett was published, I felt as though I had passed my own kind of milestone. I made an impression on myself, and I liked that feeling. It was something I had never felt before, and whatever it was that happened inside me when I wrote like that—I wanted to feel it again and again. By that point in my life, I had written dozens of college papers and an honors thesis, as well as a master's thesis. A paper I wrote about the T-4 euthanasia program in Nazi Germany was awarded $350 by a national historical honor society. As a professional communicator for the federal government, I had also written or helped write more than a hundred research reports and testimonies for Congress. But none of that writing was for *me*. What I wrote about Brett was. Writing about him and what he had confided in me was the only way I knew how to make sense of the incredible toll that keeping silent about trauma takes on those who never find a way to communicate what they survived.

When Brett recounted his stories to me—and gave me permission to write about him—he handed me a sort of power I didn't know I would crave. There was power over the story of course, but there was also power over the reader. I could use description and metaphors to make someone feel something. As soon as I learned that first piece had been accepted and was going to be published, I had this sneaking suspicion, this feeling that great and enviable things were going to start happening to me. I was going to write a book about Brett, I thought. I was going to find an agent who would sell that book for tens of thousands of dollars to a big New York City publisher, and I was going to spend months traveling the country, speaking to veterans and their families and anyone else who has ever cared about those who serve our country. I was going to save people.

My piece was published in the morning a couple of weeks before Veterans Day in 2013. The first few reader comments were positive and affirming. My friends and family shared it on social media, and before long, several people—some of them complete strangers—sent me private messages commending me for all I had done to help Brett. I saved his life, some of them said. The day after the story was published, my mother ran into Brett's mom at the grocery store, and with tears in her eyes, Brett's mom hugged and squeezed my mother for well over a minute. "Your son saved my son," she said.

A few days later, I clicked on my story and scrolled down to the bottom where the reader comments were stacking up. I skimmed through the words of affirmation as I sipped hot coffee in my home office, just down the hall from where my wife was frying eggs for breakfast.

"Go back to jerking off to Full Metal Jacket," one anonymous commenter wrote, "and leave us combat vets the fuck alone!" I put down my mug and leaned in closer to my laptop. What was this guy talking about? I couldn't understand. My hot heart pounded inside my chest as I read the rest of his rant: "Just a bunch of shitty broken vet porn," he continued, "with a bullshit ending."

I scrolled back up to the end of the story. "If it's one thing Brett has learned," I wrote, "it's that talking about your trauma can help—as long as you can find someone you trust and who helps you to take a fresh look at your experiences. While you may not be able find complete and final truths (none of us can, really), you can create meaning out of your painful experiences by creating a coherent narrative that explains them. That is what Brett has done, and it has made all the difference."

That was all true. I hadn't written anything I didn't think I would write again.

The Second Essential of Storytelling: Progressive Complications

The second essential of storytelling is what I call *progressive complications*. In this section of the story, you experience escalating degrees of conflict. If you do one thing, you'll potentially put yourself in great danger—either physical or emotional danger. If you don't, you may be tormented by regret. My progressive complication is the act of writing about Brett after he returned from Afghanistan. If I write about him, I may provoke angry reactions. I may be accused of profiting from Brett's trauma or trafficking in tragedy to fulfill some other ulterior motive. If I don't write about Brett, perhaps I may be contributing to a nationwide conspiracy to deny the reality of what war does to those who survive it.

This is the part of the story where it is appropriate to include background information and descriptions of you and your other characters. After the inciting event, once the reader is invested in the story, the reader is prepared to understand and appreciate such information. When the reader knows more about a character's history, the character's complexity elicits interest and empathy. Knowing more about a character also helps to explain the character's true motivations and frame the story appropriately. What are you holding inside and not sharing with anyone? What do you feel reluctant to disclose? Oftentimes this information is what is needed most. Just be careful not to include too much. I'm reminded of one of Kurt Vonnegut's most important rules for writing: "Every sentence must do one of two things: reveal character or advance the action."[6] In other words, there needs to be some kind of movement: either in forwarding the plot or in developing the characters.

— — —

One evening, as I was packing a suitcase for a work trip, Brett's mother, Val, texted me.

> Hi Dave I don't know if you heard but Brett was in a bad car accident last night. He will be ok but there are a lot of things involved & he may not have his job. I am worried about depression & PTSD & potentially what path he could choose. He is in Aspirus at Wausau. Thanks so much! He considers you a wonderful friend & listens to you.

> I hadn't heard.

> How long will he be in the hospital?

> ICU room 1839

What happened? Was he drunk or something?

Yes but not sure on the other details. He is lucky to be alive.

I have to go to Chicago tonight anyway. I'll pack and head up there

Concussion broken ribs & banged up.

Thanks so much!

If they move him let me know. I'll head up in 15 or 20 min

Will do!! You are a lifesaver!

Just got word from Whitney they are moving to a new room

Was he suicidal or anything? What other stuff is going on?

Not yet but extremely emotional about his job. I don't know all of details but I suspect he & Whit are having a rough time & work is all consuming

Do you know how they know he was drunk?

Blood draw at hospital.

Was he working at the time?

No although he said he was meeting an informant at a bar. He had his personal vehicle

I just talked with a lawyer friend who is a combat vet. He said department policies will dictate what happens to his career.

Thanks Dave! I appreciate that! I just keep praying since I don't know what else to do!

He's the most resilient person I know

Yes that's what gives me hope! And he has wonderful friends!

No other cars involved?

No

That's good.

He missed a corner & head on into a tree

There was no way Brett could be suicidal. He had everything he said he ever wanted. He had a loving and faithful wife who stood by him through the most difficult and harrowing times of his life. He was a hardworking and dedicated undercover drug agent for the county sheriff's office—the exact job he had wanted when he left the Marine Corps. In the first nine months of that year, Brett told me, he had racked up more drug arrests than all the other officers in the department combined. He had purpose. He had meaning. People with purpose and meaning don't wish for death.

— — —

"They said his head went through the driver-side window," Whitney told me before I entered Brett's room. She was holding her hand over her cell phone, trying to mute our conversation. Her face was puffy and pink from crying and not sleeping overnight. Her straw-colored hair was pulled back into a tight bun. She was wearing a shawl with sleeves that made her look like she was wrapped in a blanket. After she told whoever was on the phone that she would have to call them back, she hugged me tight; her face against my chest left a small tear stain on my dark-blue flannel shirt.

"You should see the other guy," Brett joked as I came into the room. His face was hard to look at. His cheeks were puffy, and the left side of his face was pocked and smeared with dried blood, which made it difficult to tell how badly the glass had cut him. From his cheekbone to his hairline, he looked like he had taken shrapnel from a grenade explosion. He chuckled and then winced in pain as I gently put my hand on top of his. Machines all around him beeped and whirred.

Brett told me he had five broken ribs and a concussion. His right middle finger had also been dislocated, and his left shoulder—the one he busted up in high school—was still out of its socket. He was in a lot of pain, and every time he wiggled or tried to get more comfortable, it felt like someone was stabbing him with a steak knife. I asked him what happened, even though I had already been told most of the details.

"I have no idea, man," Brett said. "Honestly." He shook his head and looked toward his feet at the end of the bed. He was tired.

"He was up for almost two days straight," Whitney chimed in. I hadn't noticed that she'd come back into the room. "He came home Sunday morning, tried to sleep and couldn't, so he went into town to run errands. Then one of his informants said he wanted to meet up, so Brett went to the bar to meet him."

"I had two beers with the guy," Brett said. He paused and took a labored breath. "And then I told him I had to leave. Got in the car. Don't remember anything else. I woke up here this morning."

"The state trooper said it looked like he missed a curve, went down into a ditch, and then hit a tree. The car is totaled," Whitney said.

"Were you drunk?" I asked.

"I don't know what the blood test will say," Brett replied.

He had downed a few drinks, Whitney said, but that normally wasn't enough to put him over the legal limit. "But then again," she added, "he also hadn't been sleeping or eating, so who knows what that amount of alcohol did to him?"

— — —

Brett and I spent the rest of that evening watching reruns of *American Pickers* on the small flat-screen television that hung on the wall in front of his bed. We were done talking about the accident; there didn't seem to be anything more that needed to be said. Outside the room, just within earshot, I could hear Whitney and her mother, as well as Brett's sister-in-law, talking over plans of what to do next. I tried to tune them out and focus on the television, but they were talking louder than I think they realized. It was almost as if they wanted Brett and me to hear what they were plotting.

Just as one episode was ending and another beginning, they came back into the room. Whitney stood on the opposite side of the bed as me, and Brett's sister-in-law stood at the foot of the bed, blocking Brett's view of the television. I clicked off the set as Whitney's mom sat down in a chair near the door. She clutched her purse to her chest as Brett's sister-in-law began relaying the plan.

"We talked with Josh," she said. Josh is Brett's older brother, a cop-turned-detective-turned-arson-investigator for the state. "He says you need to tell your department about your PTSD. He says you need to tell them that you were self-medicating and that you're burned out." Brett stared back at her blankly. Whitney grasped his left hand, careful not to disturb the intravenous ports.

"He says if you claim PTSD," she continued without giving Brett time to respond, "the department has to treat this accident as a medical issue. If you don't tell them, it will be a disciplinary issue, and you'll probably lose your job."

The Third and Fourth Essentials of Storytelling: The Crisis and the Climax

The third and fourth essentials of storytelling are, respectively, the *crisis* and *climax*. The crisis is the point in the story when you absolutely *must* make a decision. This decision will determine whether you'll get closer to or farther away from your object of desire, and it will reveal your true nature to the reader. How are you going to act at the moment of truth? What are you going to do? What do you *really* believe? What do you value? You must make it clear to the reader what your choices are and at least imply what the possible outcomes may be. You'll know that you've found a true crisis when it's possible that something bad could happen regardless of what decision you make. For example, let's say you're faced with the difficult decision of whether to report a wrongdoing committed by a superior at work. If you report the wrongdoing, those in authority may not do anything about it, or your peers may see you as disloyal. Or, alternatively, the wrongdoing may be stopped, and you could be seen as a hero. If you decide to say nothing, you may retain the trust and respect of your peers, although the cost of such a decision may be that someone will continue to be harmed by the wrongdoing. More than anything, the reader wants to see *how* you are going to approach and make sense of the crisis. If the decision you made was easy for you to make, then it probably wasn't a real crisis. And if it wasn't a real crisis, your reader may end up feeling cheated after sticking around for what turned out not to have high enough stakes.

The climax, in turn, is the point in the story where you actually make a decision, where you answer the question raised by the crisis. Did you report the wrongdoing, or did you look the other way? The decision you make will reveal who you are as a character to the reader. After all, actions always speak louder than words. The climax also contains the immediate result of your decision. What happened next? Keep in mind that it's not a good idea simply to allude to the decision and the immediate outcome—readers wants to see for themselves what happens.

The Fifth Essential of Storytelling: The Resolution

We all need resolution, and so do stories. How many times have you sat through a boring lecture or staff meeting and thought to yourself, *When is this thing going to end?* "A life without temporal boundaries," explains philosopher Samuel Scheffler, "would be no more a life than a circle without a circumference would be a circle."[7] The *resolution*— the fifth essential of storytelling—is about making sense of all that has happened in the story. If the inciting event shows the reader the *before*, the resolution is where the reader gets to see the *after*.

I appreciate happy endings. Not the trite, sentimental endings that mean next to nothing. Rather I'm talking about an ending where the main character is in a better place than where the character started. Everything I have done—and you have done—has been built atop everything we've lost. But that loss, that pain doesn't have to lead to cynicism or resignation. Instead, we can try to focus on how our world-views may have shifted. Did you change from a feeling of meaning-lessness to meaning? Naïveté to worldliness? Ignorance to knowing? Belief to disillusionment? Perhaps you want to focus on what you learned. Or you may want simply to tell the reader whether you got what you wanted. If you did get what you wanted, what was that like? If you didn't get what you wanted, how did you cope? If what you wanted changed, how are you now going to go about trying to achieve your new goal?

I struggled for two years to tell this story about me and Brett; I lost track of how many times I've typed it up then deleted all I had writ-ten. Time after time I would come to a certain point, and there would be no place for the story to go—except perhaps to explore the sadness of wanting things not to be the way they undeniably were. In my strug-gle of deliberation, I considered several possible endings. I could have ended the story by repeating the opening scene: Brett's going-away party at my mother's house, the night before he left for boot camp. Maybe there was a way, I thought, to extend that scene and end it with some kind of epiphany? I've heard it said that the beginning and ending of a story can be seen as mirrors hanging on opposite walls, reflecting everything that has happened in the story. How do I get my mirrors to face each other so they create the illusion of infinity? Did Brett or I say anything particularly prophetic that night that could stitch the whole story together? I cannot recall.

I also thought that perhaps the best way to end the story would simply be to tell the reader more about what all happened next. Brett resigned from his position and decided to find work that was more conducive to the less intense and middle-class life for which Whitney had waited so long. A few months after the accident, Whitney gave birth to a beautiful, healthy baby girl. They named her Josie. She looks much like Brett did as a baby. Sometime after that, Brett and Whitney sold their home and moved back to our hometown so that Whitney could open a wedding venue in an old barn her parents owned. Brett helped with the renovations and worked a series of odd-for-him jobs. He sold used cars for a little while. Then he got a job working at my father's paper mill, where he now serves as the safety supervisor. He told me not long ago that he likes the work. He punches in, works hard, and punches out. The simplicity of such a life is a breath of fresh air compared to the time in his life when he had to be armed, pretending to be someone he wasn't, and meeting informants in the middle of the night.

But where does that leave me? It is, after all, my story. Maybe I could search for subtext. Maybe I could resist the epiphany ending and describe a scene in which I walk through the hospital parking lot in the dark. I could mirror the place and time where I started to remind the reader of where I had begun my journey. I could show the reader how much had changed, and how much had stayed the same. Maybe the engine in my black Ford Escape wouldn't turn over, like the old Buick that Brett had bought off me the last year of high school.

Or maybe it would be better to focus on some theme without being too obvious. What is the point of my story? That I tried to help my friend but failed? That what first appear to be failures are really just setbacks? I could try to make this clear by focusing on sensory descriptions—smell, taste, touch, sound, and sight. I could tell the reader that it had started raining just before I left the hospital, that the raindrops were cold as they ran down my face in a stiff autumn wind, that I could smell oil and water mixing in the center of each parking space I passed. Then I could write that once I had retreated to the safety of my vehicle, I stared at my shimmery face in the rearview mirror for a minute or two before I tried to start the engine, the rain droplets falling from my beard into my lap like the tears I wish I could have shed. Such descriptions can slow down the pace of the story and bring emotional clarity without having to be explicit about what you are feeling. In my story, I was struggling to make sense of what had happened to Brett and to our friendship and what effect all that would have on my writing and my teaching. Such sensory details—which are the subject of chapter 7—also help the reader experience the situation alongside you, to feel what you feel. How could I convey my feeling of shame over having profited from, whether intentionally or not, the traumatic experiences of a friend? What would be most satisfying for the reader? I want the reader to feel something for me, but I do not want that feeling to be anger or disgust.

Another option would be to give a hint of the future. What might happen next? What does it all mean? And yet one more possibility would be to address the reader directly to say, *This is my point.*

———   ———   ———

For months after the accident, a part of me, a very vocal part, thought what that anonymous commenter wrote under my first story about Brett must have been correct after all. Perhaps I really had shoehorned a convenient ending into Brett's story. Perhaps it really *was* bullshit. Or at the very least, it had been too soon to tell what the end of Brett's story would be. By writing what I did, by wishing and hoping it were true, I felt as if I had somehow jinxed Brett. Perhaps it was because he was supposed to be "fixed"—and because everyone treated him like he was fixed and because everyone treated me like I had fixed him— that he didn't tell me he was struggling in the weeks leading up to his accident.

Putting aside all projections and conjectures, I know three things to be true. One, when Brett first confided in me that he was struggling after coming home from Afghanistan, I didn't ignore him or wish him luck or pretend that what he was experiencing wasn't as bad as he said it was. I did the only thing I could think of—I got him to write. Two, by getting him to explain what he had seen and done, I helped him reframe his experiences. Instead of focusing endlessly on what he could have done differently, Brett began to see just how much he had grown because of what he had survived. And three, it worked, or so it seemed, at least for a little while. Brett really did get better. And so did I. By helping Brett navigate his transition, I found my life's work.

I never intended that to happen, and it certainly wasn't my goal, but one thing led to another, and soon I was teaching a first-of-its-kind writing seminar for student veterans at a university in Wisconsin and getting published an edited collection of my students' stories of war and homecoming. After the book was published, I crisscrossed the country for a few years, presenting at conferences and training instructors in best practices when it comes to teaching student veterans and talking about the virtues of storytelling as a tool to help curb the appalling number of military veterans who die by their own hand. It was through these efforts that I connected with The War Horse, which hired me to be the director of writing seminars. Since spring 2017, I have continued to teach personal essay writing to military veterans and their families. What I teach helps. It empowers those who feel powerless. It brings hope to the hopeless and direction to those who feel unmoored.

But writing is not a cure-all. I know that now. For all its wondrous benefits, writing cannot prevent someone from experiencing bad days or from falling into despair. All it can do is help in the process of making sense of pain, of turning tragedy into triumph.

I also know that readers devour narratives to discover how the crisis will be resolved. Once they know, they stop reading. Let me then end with this: I wonder whether it is a mistake to dwell on all that has been lost. I wonder whether it is better instead to think about all that

Brett has given me—and what I have given him. Brett is not fixed. None of us are or ever will be. In many ways, feeling totally healed is just beyond Brett's grasp—though perhaps he is closer than he ever was before.

References

1. Michael Herr, *Dispatches* (New York: Alfred A. Knopf, 1977), 6.

2. Ty Hawkins, "Violent Death as Essential Truth in *Dispatches*: Rereading Michael Herr's 'Secret History' of the Vietnam War," *War, Literature & the Arts* 21 (2009): 129–43, http://wlajournal.com/wlaarchive/21_1-2/hawkins .pdf.

3. Julie Beck, "Life's Stories: How You Arrange the Plot Points of Your Life into a Narrative Can Shape Who You Are—and Is a Fundamental Part of Being Human," *Atlantic*, August 10, 2015, https://www.theatlantic.com /health/archive/2015/08/life-stories-narrative-psychology-redemption -mental-health/400796/.

4. Jane Alison, "Beyond the Narrative Arc," *Paris Review*, March 27, 2019, https://www.theparisreview.org/blog/2019/03/27/beyond-the-narrative -arc/.

5. Aristotle, *Poetics*, trans. Ingram Bywater, ch. 18.

6. Holly G. Miller and David E. Sumner, *Feature and Magazine Writing: Action, Angle and Anecdotes* (Malden, MA: Wiley-Blackwell, 2011), 193.

7. Quoted in Derren Brown, *Happy: Why More or Less Everything Is Absolutely Fine* (London: Bantam Press, 2016), 366.

| 6 |

Starting with One True Thing

W<small>E RAN</small> in silence as the rain fell. Steady streams of water gurgled out of dull orange drainpipes and pulsed over the edge of mildewed awnings. Further south along the seaside running path, the edge of a storm poked its beak over the roof of a weathered condo building. The rain was fat and warm, like a shower. It was my last full day on the island with my wife, and I was thankful for a break from the sensation of baking in the Okinawan sun.

Despite the endorphins coursing through my body, the thumping of a panic attack in my chest forced me to stop. Hands clasped on top of my head, I struggled to catch my breath. The blood pumped in my ears. The skin around my eyes and mouth tightened. My ribcage cinched like a belt around my lungs as I thought about all the years I had spent chasing down answers to questions about my grandfather, how far I had come, and how far away from him I still felt.

Countless hours, a few thousand dollars, and a 7,000-mile flight. All so I could retrace the route my grandfather's tank company had taken during America's longest and bloodiest battle in the Pacific theater. When I had bought the tickets, I told myself it would help me help my father better understand his father. But what I was really in search of was a story I could tell about my grandfather that didn't make me feel so ashamed of him.

— — —

Harold "Hod" Chrisinger joined the Army in the summer of 1944 at the age of 18. In a photo I have of him that was taken the summer before he joined, Hod looks much like I did when I was that age. His hair, like mine, waves from the part he combed on the right side of his head. He is crouching next to a flat tire. The car is a two-door Ford hardtop, and it is pulled to the side of a tree-lined dirt road. It's an obviously sunny day, probably around lunchtime. He is looking up with a smile that belies his predicament. With his left hand, he holds a lug wrench steady against a nut on the back left tire. With his right he is about to push. Even though the photo is black and white, I can tell his arms are as tan as they are trim. I never knew that version of him. I wish I had.

When he returned from Okinawa in the fall of 1946, he wasted little time in going back to work as a tractor mechanic in his father's shop, where he had easy access to the brown liquor served at the bar next door. It didn't take long, I've been told, for the folks around him to notice he wasn't bolted together the way he once had been.

— — —

It wasn't until years after his death that I started researching and piecing together my grandfather's story so that I could learn what had happened to him all those years ago. Just after sunrise on April 19, 1945, the tanks in his company—Company A of the 193rd Tank Battalion—along with those from the 1st Platoon from Company B of the 713th Armored Flamethrower Battalion, bobbed and weaved along a shriveled trail that would lead them up the side of a fortified ridge to their objective: a village called Kakazu. All around them, trees blended into rocks, a dirty gray smeared with green. They were supposed to flank and penetrate the rearguard of the Japanese defenses located at Kakazu, kill whatever moved, and connect with their infantry support, which was tasked with assaulting the front of the fortified ridge. Soon after arriving in the village, they realized that the infantry support wasn't coming after having been repulsed by intense Japanese fire. Without that support, the tanks were exposed and much easier for the Japanese to defeat. By late afternoon, 22 of 30 American tanks had been wiped out.

After nearly five years of on-again-off-again research, I thought I knew all the facts, but I somehow couldn't shake the feeling that I still knew nothing at all. I tried to explain this feeling to a friend of mine, an author and a veteran, who told me that if I was ever going to write anything worth reading about my grandfather, I had to go to Okinawa to see the place for myself. He said that if I wanted to really know a place, I had to feel it under my boots. And if I wanted to better understand my grandfather, I had to see with my own eyes the same ground for which he and his friends had suffered and killed.

— — —

When I sat down to write the words you're reading now, I struggled. The blank screen waited, and the cursor pulsated impatiently. I wasn't sure where to begin. What finally helped me get started, and what I believe can work for you too, is a trick that also worked for one of the most lauded writers of the twentieth century. Believing that a writer needed to have experiences to develop his abilities, a young Ernest Hemingway moved to postwar Paris. He found all the conditions there he needed for success. Not only could he live cheaply, but he could also admire the paintings of Cézanne on his way to smoky cafés where he would write each morning while sipping café crème. On days when the words wouldn't come out right—or at all—he would return to the apartment he shared with his wife, his young son, and a cat named F. Puss. Rather than berate himself for failing to do the one thing a writer is supposed to do, he would stand at the window, overlooking the roofs of Paris, and he would find calm. He had always written, he'd tell himself. And he would write again. All he had to do was write one true sentence—the truest sentence that he knew.

— — —

After two days of being let down by several battle-related tourist traps, my wife and I finally met with Jack Letscher, the amateur battlefield historian I had found through a friend of a friend. In the lobby of the hotel where my wife and I were staying, Jack surprised me with a short stack of maps he had created by tracing the path that my grandfather's company had taken during the battle. Not only was he going to take us to each battle site, Letscher said, but he was also going to show us exactly where my grandfather's tank company had been—and tell us when.

When Letscher took us to the base of Kakazu Ridge, I was struck by how different it looked from what I had imagined. It was still early in the morning, and I was already hot and sweaty as my wife and I followed Letscher across a parking lot and down a narrow sidewalk to an elevated crosswalk that arched over a busy four-lane road. The sun broiled the already red and tender skin on the back of my neck and above my elbows, where my black t-shirt could not protect me. I felt like I was finally approaching the summit of a mountain I had only dreamed of ascending.

When we reached the apex of the crosswalk, Jack pulled out a worn copy of an official military history and flipped through it until he found a map marked with a red sticky note. "Right here," he said, pointing to a topographic view of what we were now standing over. "This highway we're overlooking is the same one your grandfather's company traveled to get to Kakazu. Right under our feet. This is where they were." I felt a weight in my stomach. There's no way my grandfather, were he still alive, would recognize Kakazu Ridge today. What was once a verdant and rolling landscape was now a bustling and crowded cityscape. "And up there on top of that ridge—see that blue tower with the roof?" Letscher asked. "That's the top of the ridge. That's where the heaviest fighting took place."

"Soon after the tanks separated from the infantry," Letscher continued, "the tanks in your grandfather's company ran into a haphazard minefield, and three tanks had their tracks blown in quick succession. Stop me if you've heard all this before."

"No, it's okay," I said. "I'm here to learn."

I closed my eyes for a moment and tried to imagine what my grandfather must have experienced when he first saw this place. I thought about the living conditions inside a tank and how it must have felt like hell on earth. I could almost feel the heat from the engine. My eyes stung as I tried to imagine the smoke and the fumes. The tank's gearwheels screamed and groaned in my ears. The tracks clanked and rattled.

"After the first three tanks were disabled, the lead tank got lost in a maze of unmapped trails that snaked through here. They missed a turnoff and were ambushed by a concentration of 47-millimeter anti-tank guns that the book here says were concealed to the left of the trail they were on. They lost four more tanks that were destroyed by 16 shots. They were isolated, cut off, and couldn't spot the guns that were picking them off. That makes seven, right?" As Letscher continued, I tried to picture the antitank rounds blinking and flickering from the hills, like a faulty neon light tube.

"The remaining tanks then scurried down the road here to our right, looking for a faint track that was supposed to lead them to the village of Kakazu. They missed that turn and lost another tank to antitank fire—that's eight now."

In my mind's eye, I could see the Japanese shell, in slow motion, score a direct hit on the tank's engine, shattering the fuel tanks and starting a raging fire that spread faster than anything the other crews watching in horror could ever have imagined. I could see the clouds of billowing black smoke, mixed with licking flames, roll across the battlefield. I could see an American tanker, his face blackened and clothes alight, staggering through the smoke, eventually collapsing and rolling in agony, desperately trying to snuff out the flames.

"Then they took a wrong trail farther to the south," Letscher continued, "that led them to some relatively flat country to the east of the village."

When the tanks finally arrived on the eastern edge of the village, they found the remnants of wooden huts surrounded by once-sturdy stone walls and hedges that had been reduced to rubble by an American bombardment. Sighting through their periscopes, the gunners inside the tanks shot their 0.30-caliber machine guns at anything that moved; Japanese soldiers fell like tenpins as they emerged from their emplacements. The tanks armed with flamethrowers shot long, sticky streams of rage into cave openings and whatever buildings remained.

In addition to the official history of the battle, Letscher had brought with him a short stack of photocopied pages, with lines of text highlighted in yellow. As he read from the section he thought I'd be most interested in, a strange feeling washed over me. It felt like I had heard the words before, though I couldn't place my finger on where.

"For almost three hours," Letscher said, dragging his finger along the text, looking for the right place to dive in, "the tanks in your grandfather's company roamed back and forth through the village, blasting enemy fortifications and gun emplacements." He found what he was looking for. "Ah, right here," he said. "The tanks occupied the village, moving up and down the streets and blasting everything in sight while waiting for the infantry units to come over the ridge and join them. In this absolutely unsupported tank action, the whole village of Kakazu was utterly destroyed, and the remnants of Japanese forces were either killed or fled."

Despite a tank's tremendous firepower, without infantry support tanks were vulnerable to various forms of attack that the Japanese exploited to near perfection. In addition to antitank guns and land mines, one of the most effective methods the Japanese had for destroying an American armored vehicle was to immobilize it with a small explosive and then attack it with infantry armed with magnetic demolition charges or Molotov cocktails. If the crew came out to fight, they could be cut down by Japanese attackers at the ready. And if the crew decided instead to stay buttoned up in their disabled tank and wait for help, the Japanese would pry open the hatch and throw in grenades.

— — —

There are three kinds of first sentences: action, character, and setting sentences.

Action Sentences

Action sentences, perhaps unsurprisingly, feature action verbs. The action doesn't have to be a bomb exploding or a car speeding through a police checkpoint; it can be much simpler than that. Take, for instance, the first sentence of this chapter: "We ran in silence as the rain fell." *Ran* is the action verb, of course. "We ran in silence" puts the reader right into an unfolding event without any explanation. Writers tend to use action sentences when they want to create a little mystery. Think about my first sentence again. When you read it, you didn't know who "we" were. You didn't know why we were running (Was someone chasing us?) or why we were running in silence (Were we not speaking to each other because of an argument?). My hope as a writer was that the mystery of the action was alluring enough to hook you and convince you to keep reading.

As you know by now, I've been teaching personal essay writing for a nonprofit newsroom called The War Horse since 2017, and over the years the writing fellows I've taught in our seminars have written some really incredible opening sentences. Before I share them with you, I should note that the worksheet I use in my seminars to help writers draft their essay openers can be found in the back of this book. I should also say that some of these openers were written by people who likely would not have considered themselves writers before they attended one of my seminars. I think you'll agree that they definitely have what it takes. To start us off, here are some examples of effective action sentences:

- "A man in white appears. Above me I hear, shoot, shoot, shoot. I don't; it's my first time with a target in my sights." —Peter Lucier[1]
- "No one slept soundly."—Gretel Weiskopf[2]
- "The shopping bag lying in the street appeared harmless." —Jeremy Redmon[3]
- "'What have I gotten myself into?' I wondered while tying my shoes."—Kayla Williams[4]

- "The body was lying on an army field stretcher, nestled between the olive green metal bars, drooping lifelessly on the black mesh fabric."—Jackie Munn[5]
- "A desert butterfly perched on my leg as I rode through dusty terrain on the back end of a truck, bumping out into the desert to perform maintenance work on bombs waiting to be loaded on their jets."—Liz O'Herrin-Lee[6]

Character Sentences

A character sentence tells a brief backstory that needs to be understood about a character before the action will make sense to the reader. Instead of throwing the reader directly into the action like an action sentence does, a character sentence brings the reader close to the action by making sure that the reader knows as much as the narrator does before the action unfolds. One easy way to check whether your first sentence is an action or a character sentence is to look for adverbs of time, like *usually, always, never, sometimes, seldom,* or *often.* If your sentence includes one of these words, chances are good that you've written a character sentence that is trying to explain something about the character that the reader needs to understand above all else. Here are several examples that have been published by The War Horse:

- "There was the happy-go-lucky man I knew who laughed at everything, and then there was the man who tried to break my neck in his sleep."—Liesel Kershul[7]
- "The first time I snorted heroin felt like the peace of a sunset at dusk, the ending of the day and beginning of darkness." —Jenny Pacanowski[8]
- "Looking back, I can't help but feel responsible for my brother's decision to join the Army."—Drew Pham[9]
- "It was the last thing I had to do. The final official order of business before I could wash my hands of the whole filthy event."—Joy Craig[10]

- "Disassociation. Easily a top choice for describing my coping mechanism before age 30, and one that I can flawlessly slip back into like a favorite pair of sweatpants."—Sara Poquette[11]
- "It's an old adage among medics, that all bleeding stops. Eventually. I have to wonder now if that's true."
  —Nicole Johnson[12]

Setting Sentences

The last type of first sentence, and the trickiest to pull off in a personal essay, is the setting sentence. Setting sentences are tricky because they usually require several sentences or even a paragraph or two to get them right, and they tend to create the greatest distance between the writer and the reader. Think of it this way: The writer who begins with setting is giving readers a high vantage point from which to survey the literal and figurative landscape, but they don't generally understand what the action is, which can be hard for some readers to muddle through. When they're done well, however, setting sentences can be incredibly beautiful and poetic—almost cinematic.

The War Horse doesn't publish personal essays that begin with setting sentences all that often, but we have published a few that turned out beautifully:

- "My route took me through the plains, teeming with bugs, the heat unable to suppress the constant yet ever-changing buzzing. The sun beat down on the windswept plains, and the stalks of wheat that had bent and been warped with each gust were baked by the late summer heat."—Maggie Seymour[13]
- "A small line of people formed in front of the stage; some of them offered a handshake or a thank you, a few wanted to tell me a story about their own experience, and others asked a question or two. An older woman approached alongside a tall man who hunched at the shoulders and wore a beard that hid any expression."—Brendan O'Byrne[14]

- "The flags gently flapped in the hot breeze. The nation's colors of blue, red, and white, next to the symbol of our battalion, contrasted against the monotonous tan of the desert landscape. In front of the honor guard were a pair of polished boots, a Kevlar helmet, dog tags, and an inverted M-16 with bayonet, a somber display marking the life of Specialist Robert A. Noonan of Cincinnati, Ohio. At his service, the ranks of soldiers in their chocolate chip desert fatigues stood silently in formation as our battalion commander, the 'old man,' strode forward to honor his fallen soldier."—Harry L. Whitlock[15]

Beginning with the setting can work much better in book-length memoirs, where you have more room to play with. One of the best examples of this that I've come across is William Manchester's war memoir, *Goodbye, Darkness*, which opens with him sipping another martini aboard a Boeing 747. Decades after the end of World War II, he has decided to fly back to Okinawa to retrace the steps he took there as a young Marine rifleman during the battle:

Our Boeing 747 has been fleeing westward from darkened California, racing across the Pacific toward the sun, the incandescent eye of God, but slowly, three hours later than West Coast time, twilight gathers outside, veil upon lilac veil. This is what the French call l'*heure bleue*. Aquamarine becomes turquoise; turquoise, lavender; lavender, violet; violet, magenta; magenta, mulberry. Seen through my cocktail glass, the light fades as it deepens; it becomes opalescent, crepuscular. In the last waning moments of the day I can still feel the failing sunlight on my cheek, taste it in my martini. The plane rises before a spindrift; the darkening sky, broken by clouds like combers, boils and foams overhead. Then the whole weight of evening falls upon me. Old memories, phantoms repressed for more than a third of a century, begin to stir. I can almost hear the rhythm of surf on distant snow-white beaches. I have another drink, and then I learn, for the hundredth time, that you can't drown your troubles, not the real ones, because if they are real they can swim. One of my worst recollections, one I had buried in my deepest memory bank long ago, comes back with a clarity so blinding that I surge forward against the seat belt, appalled by it, filled with remorse and shame.

I am remembering the first man I slew.[16]

Here's another way to think about beginning your story with setting: What would a movie camera see if it started filming above the place where your story takes place and then gradually homed in on the main character? A beginning like that would be full of immersive details to help orient readers and hook them into the story. The best example I can think of to illustrate this type of beginning is Sebastian Junger's *The Perfect Storm*, which recreates a once-in-a-century storm that sank a commercial fishing vessel off the coast of Massachusetts in 1991:

> A soft fall rain slips down through the trees and the smell of ocean is so strong that it can almost be licked off the air. Trucks rumble along Rogers Street and men in t-shirts stained with fishblood shout to each other from the decks of boats. Beneath them the ocean swells up against the black pilings and sucks back down to the barnacles. Beer cans and old pieces of styrofoam rise and fall and pools of spilled diesel fuel undulate like huge iridescent jellyfish. The boats rock and creak against their ropes and seagulls complain and hunker down and complain some more. Across Rogers Street and around the back of the Crow's Nest, through the door and up the cement stairs, down the carpeted hallway and into one of the doors on the left, stretched out on a double bed in room #27 with a sheet pulled over him, Bobby Shafford lies asleep.[17]

The most important thing to remember is that an effective first sentence—or beginning to a longer story—will raise questions in your readers' minds. They will have clicked on a link to your story or opened to the first page of your book because they were curious. They wanted to know more. Once you've caught your reader's attention, that's just the beginning. The hard part is maintaining that attention in a world on fire with dings and beeps and screens and all manner of distractions. The best tool you have as a writer to keep your readers reading is to raise questions, appeal to their emotions, and then eventually answer those questions—one way or another. If you're good enough, and they find themselves hooked, they'll stick around for 20 minutes to read your story or for eight hours to read your book. If your reader cannot *feel* what matters and what doesn't, what's important and what isn't, then nothing matters. It's that simple.

— — —

About a week after Christmas, seven months after my trip to Okinawa, the doorbell rang. When I opened the door, I found a yellow envelope leaning against the storm door. Inside were a short stack of photocopied documents I had requested from the National Personnel Records Center in St. Louis, where all the remaining military personnel records from World War II are stored. Unfortunately, a fire erupted at the archives in 1973, destroying about 80 percent of all Army personnel records from World War II, including my grandfather's discharge paperwork. Of the records not destroyed, however, are more than 100,000 microfilm reels of what the Army called "morning reports." These were reports that company commanders had to fill out each morning with information about the individual soldiers under their command, including their assignments and injuries and whether any were killed in action.

I ripped open the package and flipped to the reports for April 19 and 20, 1945. There was a long list of names: the wounded, the dead, and the missing. I saw no mention of my grandfather. A week later, on April 26, the morning report updated the list of casualties: five men who had initially been listed as missing were now listed as killed in action. On April 29, another soldier's status was changed from MIA (missing in action) to KIA (killed in action). I kept flipping. On May 2, an order came for the exhausted and battle-depleted battalion to give up its tanks. Ten privates in Company A were promoted to the rank of private first class. There was still no mention of Hod anywhere.

Eighteen pages later, on May 20, I finally find mention of him: Chrisinger, Harold B., serial number 36846058. Private. His name was second in an alphabetical list of 11 other soldiers. At the bottom of the list was a typed notation: "Above eleven (11) EM atchd unasgd fr 74th Replacement Bn APO 331 per VOCO 20th Armd Gp."

What the hell did that mean?

I scanned the remaining pages, searching for corrections. I found none. Unsure of where to turn, I texted a picture of the report to a couple of veterans I know. One had been a company commander himself. Both told me it made sense: Private Chrisinger was transferred in from a replacement battalion, where he had been waiting to be assigned to an active unit in need of reinforcements. That meant my grandfather hadn't joined the company until a full month after it had been mauled in the battle for Kakazu Ridge. If that was the case, it meant he hadn't been part of the furious fighting that knocked out 22 tanks. It meant he hadn't been there that day at all. And that meant perhaps he wasn't the battle-hardened war hero I had wanted him to be.

At first, I fought it. After such an arduous journey, I couldn't accept that my grandfather had lied, that he wasn't a hero. I went back to the battalion and company records. I gathered up military maps, the pictures my grandfather had brought home with him, and every other bit of evidence I had collected over the years. I had stacks of sources printed from glitchy websites and hundreds of pages of handwritten notes on white and yellow legal pads.

As I scanned the papers, a sense of dread coursed through my veins. It was all too much. I couldn't align the dates and descriptions and testimonies. There were too many discrepancies, too many contradictions. My grandfather's discharge paperwork, for example, shows that he was inducted into the Army on August 29, 1944, and spent almost a year and a half overseas. He left for the Pacific theater on March 17, 1945, and arrived eight days later, on March 25. The Battle of Okinawa officially began less than a week after that. There is no mention of the

74th Replacement Battalion, only that he had served with the 193rd Tank Battalion. In the morning report for May 20, the day my grandfather was assigned to his unit, it says his military occupation was 2736, the Army's designation for a light tank driver. But in his discharge paperwork, his military occupation was code 050, a carpenter. Perhaps he worked as a carpenter during the occupation, helping to turn the bloody pulp of an island into a strategic launching point for the invasion of mainland Japan. Or maybe, after the bombs were dropped and the war ended, his commander wanted his paperwork to document a job that would translate better in the civilian world.

Under "Decorations and Citations," his paperwork lists (1) the Asiatic Pacific Theater Ribbon with 1 Bronze Battle Star, (2) the Victory Medal, (3) the Good Conduct Medal, and (4) the Army of Occupation Medal–Japan. Why did he have a theater ribbon with a bronze star? After a soldier's first battle, he received a theater ribbon. He would receive a small bronze battle star to be pinned to the top of the ribbon only after completing a subsequent battle or campaign. My grandfather's records seem to indicate that he participated in two battles or campaigns. But there's no other evidence that he actually did. Maybe the Army made a mistake. If so, maybe the Army made other mistakes, too. Maybe the morning report was mistaken.

I slid my fingers along the cold metal clip binding the papers and felt for a moment like giving up. My life, it seemed at that time, was like a glass tunnel, through which I had been moving faster and faster the longer I searched for answers. At the end was a mysterious darkness. After I read the morning reports, I felt like the glass had dissolved, and I was now out in the open air. Other people were suddenly closer, no longer separated from me. Ashley kept telling me that it was time to move on, that she was tired of my obsession and wanted me to participate fully in my life and in my relationship with her and in the lives of my children. She didn't want me to miss it all. She didn't want me to make the same mistakes my father and his father before him had made.

After brewing a midafternoon pot of coffee to perk myself up, I spent the next several hours transferring the language from the company and battalion records into a spreadsheet, organized by date. That way I could look at a specific date and see what the company's morning report said and compare that with what was in the battalion's "summary of action" report and its "subsequent operations" report.

Even arranged in a spreadsheet, it was still too much to take in. I thought that if I looked hard enough, it would all somehow resolve and rearrange itself into the picture I wanted to see. It didn't. After half an hour, I stood up—my knees and hips cracking as I straightened my legs—and sat with a thud on the couch. The crackly old leather pressed into my thighs. *There's nothing here*, I thought to myself. *There's nothing I can find, nothing I can say that will make any sense of this mess.* My eyes ached from the strain of scanning the blurry photocopied documents. I took off my glasses and rubbed the bridge of my nose. My journey of discovery had been one of extremes—of exhilaration and disappointment, frustration and freedom, inspiration and uncertainty, abundance and emptiness. And the vertigo of my odyssey—the unceasing contradictions, the unknowable truths—had resulted in a deep sense of melancholy. About a week later, I decided to tell my father what I had found. He didn't want to believe it. He said there must have been a mistake in the paperwork. That happens all the time, he said. He may be right. But I'm not convinced. I think Hod just lied.

—— —— ——

I'll never know if my grandfather lied because he felt ashamed by what he had done, or hadn't done, on Okinawa. The records make it clear to me that he hadn't fought in the pitched battles many of us think about when we think about World War II. Maybe he felt he hadn't faced the "Good War's" ultimate test of courage. That doesn't mean that he hadn't seen horrors—or committed them—or that he hadn't struggled and suffered.

Maybe Hod was afraid his story didn't sound like what was portrayed in the newsreels and war movies. Maybe he didn't think what he had experienced lived up to expectations of what war and heroism should look like. If that's the case, his laconic version of the ferocious tank battle may have been a sort of cover story: a version of events that was more heroic—and relatable—than an actual truth he was afraid to tell. I think my grandfather wanted his damage to be known, but for whatever reason he couldn't find the words to share the full truth. Or he simply couldn't trust that his friends and family back home would understand.

If there is a truth I can feel certain of, it is that Hod had once been a young man who went to war and that he died an old man who had never found a way to make peace with what he experienced in war. I wish he had been able to tell the truth because that's how real healing and connection take root. Instead he remained trapped alone in his cover story.

In discovering this about my grandfather, I encountered the man on a more human level: a man who was damaged and hurting—and ultimately, I feel more closeness and connection with *that* man than I could possibly have felt for an untarnished hero of the battle for Kakazu Ridge.

References

1. Peter Lucier, "My Religion of Death and Praying to Kill," The War Horse, July 5, 2016, https://thewarhorse.org/my-religion-of-death-and-praying-to-kill/.

2. Gretel Weiskopf, "The Stories I Share," The War Horse, December 18, 2019, https://thewarhorse.org/the-stories-i-share/.

3. Jeremy Redmon, "December 21 and What Came After," The War Horse, December 11, 2019, https://thewarhorse.org/december-21-and-what-came-after/.

4. Kayla Williams, "Running for My Life," The War Horse, February 12, 2020, https://thewarhorse.org/running-for-my-life/.

5. Jackie Munn, "As Iron-Filled Tears Stained the Deck," The War Horse, June 27, 2018, https://thewarhorse.org/as-iron-filled-tears-stained-the-deck/.

6. Liz O'Herrin-Lee, "Even Butterflies Go to War," The War Horse, April 18, 2018, https://thewarhorse.org/even-butterflies-go-to-war/.

7. Liesel Kershul, "Gridlock Gets You Killed," The War Horse, May 16, 2018, https://thewarhorse.org/gridlock-gets-you-killed/.

8. Jenny Pacanowsky, "Learning to Breathe through the Journey of Addiction and PTSD," The War Horse, July 6, 2017, https://thewarhorse.org/learning-to-breathe-through-the-journey-of-addiction-and-ptsd/.

9. Drew Pham, "He Craved Normalcy, but He Could Think Only of Getting Back to War," The War Horse, August 23, 2017, https://thewarhorse.org/he-craved-normalcy-but-he-could-think-only-of-getting-back-to-war/.

10. Joy Craig, "Reliving Military Sexual Trauma on Her Last Day of Active Duty," The War Horse, July 28, 2017, https://thewarhorse.org/reliving-military-sexual-trauma-on-her-last-day-of-active-duty/.

11. Sara Poquette, "Removing My Armor," The War Horse, June 12, 2019, https://thewarhorse.org/removing-my-armor/.

12. Nicole Johnson, "The Road Home," The War Horse, March 11, 2020, https://thewarhorse.org/the-road-home/.

13. Maggie Seymour, "Finding Herself on a Cross-Country Run," The War Horse, July 11, 2018, https://thewarhorse.org/finding-herself-on-a-cross-country-run/.

14. Brendan O'Byrne, "Irish Mist Adrift in the Fog of War," The War Horse, July 4, 2018, https://thewarhorse.org/irish-mist-adrift-fog-of-war/.

15. Harry L. Whitlock, "Anger Management," The War Horse, February 5, 2020, https://thewarhorse.org/anger-management/.

16. William Manchester, preamble to Goodbye, Darkness: A Memoir of the Pacific War (Boston: Little, Brown, 1979), 3.

17. Sebastian Junger, The Perfect Storm: A True Story of Men against the Sea (New York: W. W. Norton, 1997), 5.

PART III   The Story

7

Crafting Immersive Scenes

H<small>E WAS</small> stuck. Fourteen years before President Donald J. Trump issued an executive order to block immigrants from 24 predominantly Muslim countries from entering the United States for 90 days—and refugees from Syria indefinitely—President George W. Bush restricted visas for international students from Islamic states who were studying in America, using provisions afforded to him in the federal Immigration and Nationality Act.

After an 18-month background check, an Arab Muslim student named Mohamad Hafez from Syria was issued a "single entry" visa to study architecture in the United States. For eight years after the restriction was put in place by President Bush, Mohamad could not visit his family in Syria if he wanted to be able to return to his studies at Iowa State University. For eight years (until 2011), Mohamad missed weddings and funerals, holidays and boisterous family dinners. The last time he had been in the same room with his four siblings was in 2003. What had once felt like the opportunity of a lifetime became a sort of prolonged punishment.

Iowa's ruler-straight highways, melancholy summer winds, and seas of corn punctuated by small-town commercial pockets made

Mohamad long for the Barada River and the 4,000-year-old architecture of his hometown of Damascus. He missed wandering the streets of old city Damascus and sketching the ancient arches, porticoes, and doorways. He longed for the Roman city walls, the mud-brick and wood houses, and the great Omayyad Mosque. Before it was laid to waste by incessant shelling during the Syrian Civil War, Damascus was known throughout the world as a historically rich and culturally diverse city comprising Hellenic, Roman, Byzantine, and Islamic influences. Mohamad shudders to think of what it will be known for now.

To stave off the depression and intense feelings of helplessness that came from not being able to return to his home, Mohamad took the skills he was learning in his architecture courses and privately crafted Syrian streetscapes in miniature architectonic montages—from memory—out of found objects and scrap materials. He told a writer from the *New Yorker* that one evening, while he was laboring away on an architecture class assignment, he saw something he'd never noticed before. The wrapper for a Syrian chocolate he'd just eaten contained an image of the old city in Damascus. "Before he realized what he was doing," Jake Halpern wrote, Mohamad "started building a façade of an ancient wall featured on the wrapper. He worked through the night and, by morning, had completed it. In the ensuing weeks, he began churning out façades of his native city."[1] If he couldn't go home, Mohamad found he could at least re-create his home in miniature.

"My models showed my love and my passion for the multilayered culture and society of old Damascus," Mohamad told me in the spring of 2019. "In helping me deal with being separated from my family, I found catharsis and a way to celebrate the complexity and richness of the city I remembered and those that lived there."

— — —

I decided to write about Mohamad and his work after seeing one of his projects on display at the University of Chicago, where I became the director of the Harris Writing Program in February 2019. UNPACKED: *Refugee Baggage* was a small collection of what were essentially macabre dollhouses jutting out from open antique suitcases. Each miniature that Mohamad had built featured specific rooms, homes, buildings, or landscapes that had been ravaged by war and described to him by refugees from Afghanistan, Syria, or Iraq. Each miniature represented a story of loss, displacement, and devastation in an attempt to humanize refugees without romanticizing them. Passing his work each morning on my way to my office, I found the collection both beguiling and deeply unsettling, which I presume was exactly the effect Mohamad had intended.

As a teacher of public policy writing, I'm always thinking about new ways to connect with different audiences and persuade even the most steadfastly stubborn to take action. Over the past few years, I've read plenty about the Syrian Civil War in the newspaper, but I hadn't yet figured out why so much of the world seems unmoved by what's been happening there since 2011. Haven't we all seen the pictures of the bombed-out buildings and cratered courtyards? Perhaps, like me, you even cried at the images of waterlogged Syrian bodies washed up on European shores. As an American, I've worried about the troops we've sent there to fight, but at the same time, I'm ashamed to admit that before I saw Mohamad's work, I hadn't given much thought to the refugees who once called Syria home. And until I reached out to Mohamad to talk to him more about what he was trying to accomplish with his work, I hadn't delved into the psyche of someone who thought art could bridge the divide between those who are paying attention and those who are not.

The son of well-educated professionals, Mohamad is a slender man with a gentle voice. He slicks his thinning black hair straight back; it curls at the base of his neck. The horn-rimmed glasses and charcoal-gray sport coat he wears give him a thoughtful and professorial look. Beneath his smile, Mohamad grows a bushy black beard, and above it he has fashioned his mustache into amateur handlebars. "To confuse the stereotype," he told the audience that attended his artist talk at the Harris School of Public Policy in the fall of 2019.

When the Syrian Civil War erupted following the Arab Spring protests, Mohamad felt traumatized by the apocalyptic magnitude of the devastation he saw in daily news reports. "My creativity was paralyzed," he told me. "What had been my passion—my art—was cast into a block of despair. I didn't make anything beautiful for two years after that."

Once he began his career as a corporate architect, Mohamad eventually returned to his private art-making to help him process what was quickly becoming one of the worst humanitarian crises of the twenty-first century. By day, he was the lead designer for a 50-story glass and steel office tower in downtown Houston, and on nights and weekends, he made art that reflected his emotional state concerning his home country. What had begun as beautiful old Damascene façades that bounced around in his mind's eye transformed into grim depictions of the decimation wrought by modern war. "These were my artistic sneezes," he told a reporter from the *New York Times*. "If technology existed to 3-D print our emotions, my 3-D printer would make these things."[2]

— — —

"We are living in troubled times," Mohamad told me during our first interview. "Over 70 million people around the world have been displaced by war and climate catastrophe, according to the United Nations high commissioner for refugees. And on top of that, the people of Europe are agonizing about the economic and cultural impacts these millions of refugees will bring with them to their shores."

"What made you finally show your work?" I asked him, after learning that the models were not created for public consumption but were only for Mohamad himself. "Why not keep it a private form of therapy?"

"It started when I was in Italy," he explained. "I was there procuring marble for my project in Houston, and I got a call from my brother-in-law. 'I'm in Sweden,' he tells me. 'Can you come here?'"

The war and the destruction and the mass migrations suddenly overwhelmed Mohamad. "It felt like I had flown straight into a concrete barrier," he said. "Seeing my brother-in-law in that refugee camp with other refugees from all over the world—it looked like the UN or something—I started to think that perhaps my art could be useful in connecting people in these deeply divided times."

How to Write with Immersive Details

When I sat down to write a reflection on Mohamad's work, I knew I needed to find small but significant details to bring him to life—just as he routinely does in his own meticulously detailed work. I started my search by reading several profiles of Mohamad that had already been written. Then I interviewed him myself, of course, first over the phone and then in person. I also attended an artist talk he delivered. During my first interview with him, I asked him what he thought about when he worked, what his motivations were. I found pictures of him, his work, and his studio, and I asked what he saw, heard, and smelled while he was working. My goal from the beginning was to sketch out a story structure and then fill in that structure with immersive and evocative details so that I could make readers feel or sense something specific without having to state flatly what I wanted them to feel. If a detail or quote didn't illuminate, I left it out. If it did not show the reader something specific and important about the situation, I got rid of it. Famed horror writer Stephen King describes this skill of illumination in writing as making the reader "prickle with recognition."

As I began fleshing out the Five Essentials of Storytelling and weaving together the details I uncovered in my reporting, I was reminded of an experience I had during college. The lights were dimmed when I entered a small studio. My classmates were sharpening pencils with pocketknives, flipping their enormous pads of drawing paper to a clean sheet, or adjusting the height or angle of their easels. Life Drawing I was the first time we would be drawing a live nude model. My pulse quickened when the model entered the studio from the supply closet in the back of the room. It wasn't the anticipation of university-sanctioned nudity that brought on my anxiety but rather anticipation

of the eventual moment when the model would stroll among us bud-
ding artists, glimpsing at what we had drawn.

With my charcoal pencil at the ready, the young woman—we were
not told her name—dropped her thin white robe to the floor, stepped
out of the rumpled pile at her feet, and struck a pose in the center of
the room. She placed her left hand on her narrow hip, her left elbow
jutting out from her side. She placed her right hand at the base of her
neck and tilted her head backward. The vent overhead was gently
moving air; I could see it in her long brown hair, which hung loose
down to the middle of her back. Soon the sound of pencil tips scraping across thick paper filled my ears. "Five minutes," the professor
boomed over the noise. "Focus on the form. Capture a strong sense of
the pose. Don't overwork the drawing. Keep things simple. Save the
details for last."

The dim lights in the ceiling shining down on her arms cast dark,
crisp shadows across her torso. Her bare legs looked stiff, locked at the
knees. Below her muscular thighs she had bony ankles and feet. One
foot, her left, was pointed straight ahead, straight at me. The other
was open, pointing 90 degrees from the left.

Once her pose was set, I measured the length of her torso with my
pencil by extending my arm straight in front of me. I closed my right
eye and used my pencil to gauge the distance between where her neck
ended and her legs began. Then on my page I separated the measured
torso into rib cage, abdomen, and hips. After that, it was time to mark
the openings of her limbs and group her major muscle groups using
simple forms.

At the end of the first minute, I was drawing simple ovals to add
muscles and indicate where her kneecaps and elbows were positioned.
Having her left foot pointed straight at me foreshortened her leg from
my vantage point, which I needed to account for to ensure that the figure I was drawing was more three-dimensional on the page. I did this
by emphasizing overlaps. Giving myself lots of chances to get it right,
my pencil passed over the paper quickly, the charcoal marks piling up
fast. Sketch and layer. Sketch and layer. Next I turned to her muscles

and emphasized the parts where they overlapped, which further created the illusion of life through detail.

Faces have always given me the most trouble, so I saved hers for last. Most of what I could see was the underside of her chin and the hollow emptiness of her nasal passages, so I started with her jawline. We all know that a jaw curves at a certain angle, but everyone's jaw is slightly different in a thousand tiny ways. If you get that curve wrong, nothing about the drawing will look quite right. *How was her jaw unique?* I asked myself as I sketched and layered. What is the tilt? And the rotation? Where are the shadows and lines of muscle on her neck? I tried to capture what I could see of her hairline and the way the light fell across her face. *Draw the darkest darks first,* I thought—a lesson my mother had taught me.

"One more minute," the professor announced.

With what little time I had left, I ignored the details in her hands and feet and focused instead on the unique tilt in her hips, the slope of her shoulders, and the gracefulness of her collarbone. Would her friends or family be able to recognize her? What did her pose, unprompted by the professor, tell me about who she was? Was she projecting warmth? Defiance? Delight?

Long before I ever considered myself a writer, I had learned to notice the details that make a person imperfect and unique and distinctive and beautiful. Such details, when I found them in Life Drawing I, were what made a drawing feel real. Such is also true for our stories that need to be told: details matter. When it comes to details, writers need to be specific like visual artists are, and the best way I have found to be specific is to *show* the reader what you experienced.

Mohamad's work is a perfect example of this. When he interviewed refugees about their experiences, he said that his ears usually perked up whenever interviewees vividly described something or used a specific name for what they were re-creating in their mind's eye. His ears also perked up whenever he heard interviewees use strong verbs of action or when they used metaphors, similes, or other forms of figurative language. (A metaphor is a figure of speech that describes something in a way that isn't literally true but that helps explain its nature, and a simile is a figure of speech that compares one thing to another). When interviewees spoke about something in this way, Mohamad knew what they were describing was particularly impactful for them. He got especially excited whenever an interviewee described a smell, which may be the most underrated of all the senses a writer can appeal to. After all, an imaginative description of a smell can fill a reader's nostrils, waft through their gray matter, and dust off blurry memories that bring them much closer emotionally to the writer.

To be clear, the writer's goal is not simply to record as many details as possible. That would leave nothing for readers to imagine for themselves. Instead, Mohamad told me, the goal should be to find a handful of immersive details that reveal the true essence of a character or scene.

In an essay by writing fellow Brendan O'Byrne, who attended the first seminar I taught for The War Horse, he describes an older woman he met after a book signing. His description does a wonderful job, I think, of revealing the character's true essence: "Light blue specks of splattered paint polka-dotted her pair of faded jeans. She wore a light-colored fleece and thick-framed reading glasses. She had aged kindly. The corners of her eyes and mouth wrinkled to show years of smiles and laughter. It seemed like some of those small lines were damp. Gray streaks highlighted her black hair."[3]

Without much telling, Brendan shows us what this woman looked like and allows us to draw our own conclusion about her. When I read this, I see a working-class woman. Maybe she's self-employed. A house painter perhaps. She's from a small town or a rural area, like the place where I grew up. Perhaps her son or someone else she was close to had joined the military after 9/11—that's why she had been crying and had come to the book reading in the first place. What she lacked in wealth, however, she made up for in warmth and kindness. That sounds a lot like many of the people I grew up around.

The way something sounds—or even simply naming the sound—can be another powerful detail to include in your writing. Drew

Pham, for example, wrote these descriptive lines in a haunting essay: "In that damp malt and hops perfumed basement, we were encircled by military-aged youth nodding and shifting to the singer's hoarse screams, the vibrating guitars, the machine gun rattle of the drums."[4] Another former student of mine, Yvette M. Pino, used interesting verbs and descriptions of sounds to create a sense of foreboding in her account of a time she and some other soldiers were locked in a bomb shelter during an artillery attack in Iraq: "There came a dull screech, and the knuckled moan of metallic hinges bearing too much weight slowed time. I heard the pin rotate, the reverberating verification that open was now closed."[5]

As for the other senses, describing the taste of something bad can make a reader recoil as though they too have tasted it. The same goes for touch. If you describe something pleasurable to touch, your reader will experience pleasure. If you make it painful, the reader will wince in pain.

While learning more about how Mohamad picks up on the immersive details he tries to capture in his work, I heard the story of Amjad, a Syrian refugee Mohamad interviewed in Connecticut. During the early days of the Arab Spring, Amjad became an activist, marching in one of the first antigovernment protests. He saw friends killed; others disappeared. He hated the Syrian secret police, which were known to him and his friends as Al Shabeha—"the ghosts." The anger and fear Amjad felt toward them bubbled to the surface every time he saw a white Peugeot 504. In addition to being a midsize, front-engine, four-door sedan, the Peugeot 504 is also the Syrian secret police's car of choice. For Amjad, the car itself became a trigger for a terrible memory that clicks into place in his mind every time he thinks of one. What he remembers is that he saw a white Peugeot 504 parked down the street from his house one day. Black-clothed armed thugs occupied the two front seats. In the back was his handcuffed neighbor, a fellow activist. The car left shortly after Amjad had spotted it. In an effort to earn their son's release, his neighbor's parents sold nearly all their possessions so they could afford the payment demanded of them. Soon after they made the payment, the son's cold dead body was delivered to his parent's front door without explanation or justification.

— — —

I can imagine Mohamad in his studio crafting this scene from Amjad's life back in Syria. The air smells of incense and strong Syrian coffee. Tranquil notes of traditional Syrian music play softly in the background. On one of the walls is 15 feet of stacked shelves bearing the weight of all manner of broken appliances large and small, discarded piano keys, jars of old paintbrushes, busted radio components, wires, and other random bits of other people's trash. On the opposite wall hangs a series of works in progress—replicas of half-destroyed apartment complexes hemorrhaging electrical wires and rusted pieces of metal rebar. The cleanest, tidiest of all the replicas is the one inspired by Amjad's story.

There are no crumbling shafts of concrete or other evidence of bombs or bullets. There is but a stone wall looking centuries old, made of a slab of foam painted intricately to resemble weathered concrete and plaster. The wall's faded turquoise and ocher patina evoke better times now gone for good. What to an untrained eye would appear to be mismatched brass and copper ornaments become, for Mohamad, an ancient-looking doorknob to Amjad's neighbor's front door. A malfunctioning Christmas bulb was whispered to new life as a solitary streetlight hanging above a miniature sidewalk. There are no people. The effect is ghostly and unnerving. Most sinister of all, a child's toy car is now a symbol of oppression and brutality after Mohamad affixed to it miniature government license plates. The tiny scene, with its high-fidelity design, forces viewers to squint and take a step closer until they're practically inside the haunting world Mohamad created from discarded trash.

The stunningly real details in Mohamad's work are what stick with you long after you've left the exhibit. The details are what form connections for the viewer to the subject and what make the skin on your arms tingle and your knees feel wobbly. The details, most of all, are what have given Mohamad some semblance of peace. "My soul is deeply troubled," he told the *New Yorker*, "witnessing everything that has happened in Syria. I don't talk much. I don't go to therapy, but my emotions want to yell out. And I cannot console myself in anything other than this highly detailed work."[6]

References

1. Jake Halpern, "An Artist's Obsession with the Ruins of His Homeland," *New Yorker*, April 4, 2017, https://www.newyorker.com/culture/culture -desk/an-artists-obsession-with-the-ruins-of-his-homeland.

2. Brett Sokol, "A Little Piece of Downtown Damascus in New Haven," *New York Times*, October 12, 2017, https://www.nytimes.com/2017/10/12/arts /design/mohamed-hafez-syria-new-haven.html.

3. Brendan O'Byrne, "Irish Mist Adrift in the Fog of War," The War Horse, July 4, 2018, https://thewarhorse.org/irish-mist-adrift-fog-of-war/.

4. Drew Pham, "He Craved Normalcy, but He Could Think Only of Getting Back to War," The War Horse, August 23, 2017, https://thewarhorse .org/he-craved-normalcy-but-he-could-think-only-of-getting-back-to-war/.

5. Yvette Pino, "Unclear All-Clear and a Requisite for Air," The War Horse, June 13, 2018, https://thewarhorse.org/unclear-all-clear-requisite-air/.

6. Halpern, "Artist's Obsession with the Ruins of His Homeland."

8

Using Fiction to Tell the Truth

MEMOIR IS not courtroom stenography. All storytelling, whether it's memoir or not, is art. And all art is imagination, projection, and performance. The imagination comes when you mentally glide backward into the past to reencounter an experience. Projection occurs once you dig into that experience and try with great specificity to record what you thought and felt at the time. The performance, of course, is in the telling.

What do you do, though, when the past you want to explore can't actually be explored?

You could lie.

For several years before I wrote this book, I wanted to lie about my grandfather to anyone who was willing to listen. I wanted to tell a story, a fiction, about how he couldn't wait to turn 18, how he signed on Uncle Sam's dotted line in a fit of wholesome, patriotic fervor. About how he was a spirited and motivated all-American boy who was highly trained and exceedingly principled, who only ever did what he had to do to survive. About how he never took pleasure in the pain and suffering of others. About how he wanted nothing more than to come home, raise a family, build a business, and take his rightful place among America's Greatest Generation.

Most of that isn't true, as you know. I decided not to lie about him after all, because I realized that from a reader's perspective, a character's failures and shortcomings and weaknesses are the most interesting things about him. Those are the things that make us relatable. Those are the things that make us human.

If you're going to be a memoirist, you cannot lie to yourself—or to anyone else. You could write fiction instead; just don't call it a memoir.

Here's some more truth that you're now well aware of: I don't actually know all that much about what my grandfather experienced during the Battle of Okinawa. He didn't like to talk about his war, and he died before I could work up the courage to ask him about it. For decades after he came home, the details of what he experienced came out in fragments, here and there, leaving in their wake only tension and puzzlement, shame and confusion.

After I published a short essay about my journey to uncover the truth in the *New York Times'* At War column, I received hundreds of emails and comments from readers who either felt connected to what my family had experienced and wanted to share with me their own stories of tension and puzzlement, shame and confusion, or who had a different perspective on what could have happened to my grandfather—and what it meant. For example, a former Marine intelligence officer who was stationed on Okinawa in the early 1980s wrote, "If it's any consolation, I believe there is only a 50% chance your interpretation is correct regarding your grandfather's participation in the Okinawan battle timeline." He said that he had always been a history nerd and had spent lots of time while stationed on Okinawa going through morning reports and records of the battle. "You should take that morning report with a grain of salt," he continued. "In the chaos and fog of war, replacements were frequently sent in willy-nilly, and without any paperwork." The bottom line, he wanted me to know, is that "the date of the report is not necessarily the day the event happened, merely the day it was reported to the admin clerk for logging. In many cases, replacements were already dead before they had even officially checked in or the paperwork showing their new unit attachment caught up to them."

Another reader, a doctor who had spent much of his career trying to understand and explain how "responsible men, family men, churchgoing men, regularly turn into monsters throughout history," told me simply that, based on his research, my grandfather may not have lied intentionally. "Memory is not reliable," he wrote. "We reshape it to fit all manner of influence, not just internal thoughts, but external voices, particularly the constant retelling by others."

He's right. Our brains recall memories with a different wiring than when we verbalize what we remember. Once the memory is conveyed to a reader or a listener in the form of a story, it's nearly impossible for us not to rearrange and shorten and emphasize certain parts over others. We reconstruct, fill in holes, and add our own personal flourishes, forever tarnishing the "purity" of the original memory. And in the case of a traumatic experience, stress hormones rush memories to the nonverbal limbic centers of our brains, which is why we experience traumatic events so viscerally and why traumatic memories are frequently choppy and disjointed. In nontraumatic situations, the hippocampus is responsible for transiting short-term memory to verbal, long-term storage areas of the brain. What is written or spoken, for better or worse, becomes textured and dramatized.

Some other readers wondered what he might have experienced in the last few weeks of the war—I wonder that, too—and one reader in particular accused me of cherry-picking the worst of my grandfather's postwar behavior to disparage his service. "The Battle of Okinawa lasted almost a full month after the May 20 transfer," the reader pointed out. "If the grandfather was on Okinawa for that 29 days, he had to see a lot of action. He answered the call, he did not obviously shirk his duty in an area of heavy battle and he returned home. Enough said on that score. His other later problems could have other causes.

Not every vet was a good guy and the service was not automatically to blame."

"Why demean your grandfather for his exaggerations about his military service?" another reader asked. "He had nothing else in his life that he felt he could be proud of. Some people are so inarticulate that they can only maintain a fiction that he would have loved to experience. We all lie to ourselves."

While the personal essay and memoir are the cornerstones of creative nonfiction and are, by definition, concerned with telling the truth, the real truth is that we all lie to ourselves. I lie. And so do my students. In the essays they write, almost everyone massages the truth about things they've done and things they haven't. Sometimes intentionally, other times not. Either way, each one of us continually renovates memories in an effort to create stories in our own heads that bring coherence to chaos.

During the past decade of teaching writing to trauma survivors, I've heard lots of what I think may be tall tales. Sometimes my students haven't made sense of their trauma and their memories about it, and massaging the truth, whether consciously or not, can be therapeutic. The style of personal essay I teach gives writers the chance to try out narratives, to see how they fit, and to see how others react to them. I've seen time and again that this process of turning their lives and experiences into a coherent story—is hugely important to a survivor's journey to wholeness.

It doesn't bother me that my students' stories might not be completely true. I recognize and appreciate that the chemistry and mechanics of a human brain make it exceedingly difficult for a survivor of trauma to know *exactly* what happened. I recognize that the world is full of complexity and fracture and ambiguity and contradictions and that the particulars of a memory aren't always essential. What's much more important is that each of us finds a way to live with the story we tell ourselves. And when the past you want to explore cannot easily be explored, you'll need to use a combination of memory, knowledge, research, observation—and sometimes a little imagination, too. The most important thing is that you're transparent with your readers about when you're doing what. If you're not sure something happened exactly as you remembered it, tell them that. If you're imagining or speculating, be honest about it. It should be our goal as storytellers, above all else, to make our readers believe us, to hit the same notes we once felt deep inside when we experienced the truth for ourselves.

Some truth, you'll find, sits more heavily in the gut. For all we do not know about my grandfather's wartime experiences, what we do know is that he claimed to have experienced traumas and rude awakenings, though surviving a disastrous tank battle likely wasn't one of them. His trauma came from other things. Chief among them, I believe, was the way he and the other soldiers in his platoon had treated Japanese prisoners at the tail end of the battle. His rude awakening was an awakening to the fact that war required an eroding of the veneer of civilization, that war made a savage of him and his friends, that, to survive, he would need to exist in an environment totally incomprehensible to anyone back home in Wisconsin.

There was a story he told my father once, years and years ago, about a prisoner of war. The first time my father relayed this story to me, he said it was a young Japanese soldier who had surrendered to my grandfather's platoon. The second time he told me the story, it was a young Okinawan boy, a conscript, who had been captured after trying to throw a grenade toward a squad of patrolling soldiers. Maybe it doesn't matter all that much whether the man was Japanese or Okinawan, or whether he surrendered peacefully or was captured. We don't have to know the particulars of history in order to know it in our bones. The point of the story was that my grandfather had, according to his version of events, been too soft with this prisoner. The way he told it, he felt bad for the boy. Both the boy and my grandfather were nothing more than scared kids. Maybe that realization caused my grandfather to drop his guard. Maybe he wasn't as menacing as he needed to be. Whatever it was, my grandfather's platoon leader, tense faced and nerve racked, chewed his ass in front of everyone—even threatened to shoot my grandfather if he didn't start treating the enemy like the cunning bastards he believed they were.

—— —— ——

The reader comments I took most seriously were from those who didn't seem to appreciate my compassionate response to my grandfather's lie and his years of suffering with addiction. One reader accused me of whitewashing his abusive relationship with my grandmother. "I think the author wants, or needs, to believe his grandfather was a good man who had a blip of cruelty," one reader wrote, "and he's trying desperately to assemble that proof for himself and his father. The likely truth is that the grandfather was a bad person who became kinder when age and frailty forced him down from his throne."

Maybe so.

"The story of his abuse of your grandmother already told us he wasn't a hero," another reader commented. "Many abusers are liars about their history. Now you know what everyone should know: there is no excuse for becoming an abuser."

One reader in particular, a woman named Patrice, had such a strong reaction to my essay that she not only wrote a letter to the editor of the *Times* expressing her displeasure, but she also emailed me a copy of what she had written. "In detailing the lengths to which he went to try to make a batterer into a battered war hero," she began, "David Chrisinger has inadvertently provided a case example of the generational transmission of male supremacy. Even after discovering that his grandfather not only abused his family but also lied about his military record, Chrisinger showers him with sympathy for presumed harms suffered during his service.

"For the record," she continued, "PTSD does not compel men to shove their wives' faces into toilets. Such acts are motivated by misogyny and a presumption of privilege. Such deep-seated feelings of antipathy and superiority are not created by a few years away at war, although they may be compounded by it. Instead of continuing to try to find excuses for abusive behavior, I hope that Chrisinger spends at least as much time learning his grandmother's story, including but not limited to the trauma she endured at the hands of his grandfather, as he did trying to make her batterer into a hero."

My grandmother's story absolutely does need to be told. And someday I will tell it. I promise you that, Patrice.

—— —— ——

George David Chrisinger was born 7 pounds, 13 ounces on July 13, 2011, in Alexandria, Virginia. He was a day late and a little jaundiced. Ashley and I spent two nights in the hospital with him, barely sleeping at all. Between the frequent feedings and the pleather recliner reserved for sleepy fathers, neither one of us found much comfort.

While I was packing up our belongings, just before we were discharged, one of the nurses came into our room to see if we needed anything. I told her we were fine. She smiled and said there was one thing she wished someone would have told her when she brought her first child home. "If you can," she said, "sleep when the baby sleeps. It's the only way to keep yourself from going insane the first few weeks."

George was a dreadful sleeper. During the first few days at home, I don't think he slept more than 45 minutes at a time. The air inside our one-bedroom apartment just off the interstate was thick and muggy; our window unit couldn't keep up with Virginia's July weather. For the most part, I felt entirely useless. Ashley didn't want him using bottles, and nothing I did seemed to comfort him. The first time I tried to change his diaper in the middle of the night, I forgot to place a wet wipe over his crotch, and as I bent down to grab a fresh diaper, a warm stream of urine shot through the darkness, blasted me in the forehead, and dribbled down my face.

The next day, I tried something different. Instead of impatiently rocking George in my arms, upset at myself for my inability to soothe him, I lay on our leather sectional with him snuggled on top of my bare chest under a blanket. His wrinkly ear pressed to my heart, and with his tiny yellow fingers, he combed the tuft of hair in the center of my chest until he drifted off to sleep without a fuss. I breathed deeply, from the stomach, like a rancher trying to tame a wild horse. I needed him to feel that I was calm and that I was safe and that he too should feel safe. Soon enough, his breathing matched my own rhythm, albeit at a faster pace. I remember wondering, in the stillness of that small triumph, whether my father had ever held me that way and whether he and I would ever have any time for each other again.

Twelve days after George was born, my grandmother passed away at Gunderson Lutheran Medical Center in La Crosse, Wisconsin. She was 85 years old. When I asked my father whether he'd be able to pick me up at the airport if I found a last-minute ticket from DC, he told me not to worry about coming. He knew money was tight for us, and he wanted me to be there for my wife and new son. George won't be little forever, he reminded me. He seemed to be in a healthy place of acceptance, and I reassured myself that he probably didn't need me to be there for him. I thanked him for his understanding and told him to give the rest of our family my best. If I'm honest with myself, I was relieved not to be guilt-tripped into traveling home for the funeral. While I would miss my grandmother, her loss was not a devastating one for me. I loved her, but I also didn't feel as connected to her as some of her other grandchildren did.

I learned much more about her in the years after her death, when I started learning more about my grandfather's story. I feared I wouldn't be able to handle whatever grief I'd be exposed to at the wake and funeral. The underlying silence of grief suffered at the death of a loved one—the frightened and recessive grief—had always been too much for me. Perhaps my fears were unfounded. Years later, my father told me that unlike when his father passed, he was ready for his mother's death. She had finally found peace, he told me. It was her time. "Failure to thrive" was her official cause of death, though I'm sure the emphysema, heart disease, and pneumonia certainly didn't help her "thrive."

My grandmother's obituary said that she was a homemaker and a wonderful cook and that she enjoyed caring for her family. All that was true, I suppose. What it didn't say was that she was an orphan who had found her father dead after he swallowed rat poison to spare himself the grief he felt after his wife had died from a postsurgical infection. It also didn't mention that my grandmother had been the wife of a drinking man for nearly four decades and that her life, though full of as much love as she could muster, had been simple and small and hard. I wish whoever had written the obituary would have mentioned that she had a way of making others feel important and loved and that despite all she endured, she had raised well-mannered and hardworking children whose lives, thankfully, ended up entirely different from her own.

In the early 1940s, everyday life in America was characterized by an underlying condition of peril where self-restraint, reticence, temperance, and wariness were necessary to minimize the inherent risks. Profound suffering was never too far off for most. The adults my grandparents grew up around surely had a moral abhorrence for anything that would make life even more perilous, which probably contributed to my grandparents' decision to tie the knot on April 6, 1944, not long after they had to come clean about my grandmother's pregnancy.

My father's older sister, Mary, told me that when my grandmother was a teenager, before she got pregnant, she had a crush on a boy named Raymond Olsen, the man she would later marry after leaving my grandfather. Perhaps she might have married him instead of my grandfather the first time around were it not for the bachelor uncles my grandmother lived with outside of town. After her father committed suicide, my grandmother and her youngest brother moved in with these two uncles, and my grandmother raised her little brother, cooked, and cleaned. They told her Hod was the better catch and that she should marry him, not Ray. The effects of the Great Depression were still being felt all around them, and Hod's family was relatively wealthy. Unlike most other teenagers in town, my grandfather always had new clothes to wear and relatively new cars to drive. He didn't want for anything. He was handsome, too. Or perhaps that was just the story my grandmother told to make sense of her pain and disillusionment. No one can be sure. It's entirely possible that my grandparents, like many couples of that era, had simply been children together and matured together. Perhaps such closeness had produced in them love's illusion.

When my grandfather left on a train bound for San Francisco, where he would board a battered troop ship headed west across the Pacific, my grandmother moved out of her uncles' farmhouse and into my great-grandparents' home. Mary told me that my grandmother didn't get along with my great-grandmother, Maude. When I asked why not, she said that Maude didn't think my grandmother was good enough for her son. Having my grandmother move in with her and my great-grandfather, Harry, was Maude's way of "doing her part" for the war effort, she said.

In addition to keeping a close eye on my grandmother and thwarting whatever effort she might have put into running around on my grandfather while he was overseas, Maude also took to indoctrinating my grandmother, with the help of the leading ladies' magazines of the day, about her role and responsibilities as they related to my grandfather if and when he returned from the front. It was, after all, the wife's or girlfriend's responsibility—according to these publications—to make her man's transition back to family life as smooth as possible. With a new baby to care for and few educational and economic prospects, my grandmother found herself in the grip of something that wouldn't let her go.

—— —— ——

Sometimes I feel compelled to invent scenarios, to fill in the holes of half-told stories. I picture the magazines lying on my great-grandmother's living room coffee table, curated and archived after her brother was killed in Tunisia and after she realized that, unless the war ended in 1944, her son was probably going to be called as well. I picture Maude picking through the pile, looking for the dog-eared pages of an article she knew my grandmother needed to read.

"The truth is that women's work begins when war ends, begins on the day their men come home to them," Dorothy Parker wrote in Vogue. "For who is that man who will come back to you? You know him as he was. . . . But what will he be, this stranger who comes back? How are you to throw a bridge across the gap that has separated you—and that is not the little gap of months and miles?"[1]

One woman named Stella, who was married to a "victim of combat fatigue" named Ed Savickas, threw her bridge across the gap by dedicating herself to meeting her husband's fluctuating needs, routinely and discreetly. In an article published in *Ladies' Home Journal*, Stella was praised for her unwavering devotion. "The best thing for returned cases of combat fatigue," the author wrote, "would be to supply each guy with a wife like Stella, aware that merely loving your guy isn't enough to help him get squared round."[2]

Other writers didn't go quite as far. The key, one noted in *Good Housekeeping*, was to realize that, "After the euphoria of homecoming[,] . . . your husband may begin to feel let down. He may become aware of the years he has lost, of the job he left, of the bright future he abandoned, of the insecurities that lie ahead." He might be depressed "after the first thrill of homecoming has passed" because men who have lived through the bitter and harrowing experiences of war are almost always depressed, as though, "after the relief of their own escape has worn off, they feel almost guilty that they lived while others died." The solution was not to push a man out of his funk or to shame him. Instead, a good wife was supposed to "encourage him to talk the experience out, or even cry it out. He will, in a sense, be going through a period of mourning."[3]

In May 1945, soon after the Germans surrendered, Irene Stokes Culman wrote an article for *Good Housekeeping* with a title that didn't mince words: "Now Stick with Him." The year the war ended was a banner one for divorce in the United States. More than 500,000 marriages ended that year—about 31 for every 100—and by 1947, the United States had the highest divorce rate in the world, doubling its prewar rate. That was simply unacceptable to Irene Stokes Culman. Throwing a bridge across the gap that formed during the war was going to take time, patience, and compromise, she wrote—"lots of it, probably years and years. To him, undoubtedly, you seem very different, too. He has his own adjustments to make, in all likelihood much greater than yours." A little stick-to-itiveness couldn't hurt, either. "You took your soldier, young woman," Culman concluded with a distinctly matriarchal tone. "He's yours. In heaven's name stick with him."[4]

The message was clear. Ignore the disturbing behaviors. Don't take them personally. Life may not pick up where it left off. No man, after all, can go through the grim business of war and come home emotionally intact. There will be problems. There will be setbacks. Be prepared. Don't give up.

Though our views on marriage and gender equality may have grown more progressive in the generations since, our assumptions and reductive fears about the returning soldier have barely evolved at all.

— — —

On May 1, 1945, my grandfather's tank battalion had its remaining tanks taken away and distributed to better-performing battalions on the island. From that point until the end of the summer, his company was tasked with completing the often-forgotten final phase of the battle—mopping up whatever Japanese resistance remained in the central lowlands of the island. On May 19, according to his battalion's operations report, my grandfather's company, along with Company B and a reconnaissance platoon from the headquarters company, were tasked with "sealing caves" and the "cleaning out of enemy civilians and military personnel." The captain who typed up the report claims that they encountered no military personnel but that thirteen "enemy civilians were apprehended and turned over to military authorities, and a total of forty-one caves were closed in the area."

On June 5, a motor patrol from my grandfather's company picked up three civilians and turned them over to military policemen at Camp Hiza. Four days later, a patrol from the same company was sent to the towns of Chibana and Nishibaru to investigate a report of unauthorized civilians "operating" in that area. Several unoccupied caves were encountered and sealed, but no civilians were located. Then, on June 21, a patrol from Company A was sent to sweep a gully and encountered two enemy soldiers. Both were killed. There were no

American casualties reported. Four days later, after a camp guard killed two enemy soldiers lurking near the civilian camp at Koza, a large patrol from my grandfather's battalion swept the area around the camp and apprehended 15 young Okinawan men who were then handed over to military policemen at Camp Koza.

Patrolling a hostile land, even after the worst of the fighting had ended, was still no picnic. It was even worse for soldiers who, like my grandfather, never received much training in small-unit tactics. Toward the end of the war in the Pacific, losses had been so great that men who were woefully unprepared for combat were being flung without hesitation into its raging furnace. By the time Allied forces invaded Okinawa, American replacements could expect only a scant 60 days of training, some as little as six weeks. Life expectancy for a replacement could be, as a result, relatively brief.

Some of my veteran students explained to me once that going out on patrol and fighting the enemy were two totally different experiences. In direct combat, fear normally moved swiftly. It struck hard at first and then oozed away as training and muscle memory took over. Shots were fired. Grenades thrown. People screamed like mad. Then it was over faster than it had begun. As long as there was action, soldiers didn't have much time to be frightened. But on patrol, fear was slow burning, heavy, and stomach filling. All movement was careful and slow. Crablike. That's the same way pain can work, too—slow.

In the years I've spent researching my grandfather's story, I've never come across a history of the Battle of Okinawa that explained what it was like to engage in such a tough, methodical grind to wipe out the last remaining pockets of Japanese soldiers-turned-guerillas. The pitched and bitter skirmishes waged in countless caves and gullies—punctuated by encounters with frightened and emaciated noncombatants—did not make the front pages of newspapers back home. It makes sense; no war correspondents seemed to have tagged along for the grisly ride. Those newspaper editors and the folks back home had already turned their attention to the next battle, the invasion of the mainland of Japan. The mud-smirched, unshaven soldier killed here or there clearing a cave of civilians wasn't nearly as news-worthy as the 1,656 Marines who died fighting for Sugar Loaf Hill or the nearly half a million GIs who were expected to become casualties when they landed on Kyūshū, the southernmost Japanese island. Another thing that didn't make the news and apparently wasn't worth mentioning in the popular histories was the barbed-wire "relocation camps" that American troops built to house the thousands of "enemy civilians" who called Okinawa home.

I wonder if my grandmother ever read Edgar L. Jones's *Atlantic Monthly* essay, which was published after the war ended but before my grandfather returned from the Pacific. I suspect not, although I wish she had.

"What kind of a war do civilians suppose we fought, anyway?" Jones asked. As a former soldier in the British Eighth Army, army historian, and war correspondent who covered the battles of Iwo Jima and Okinawa, Jones had personally witnessed American soldiers and Marines in both Europe and the Pacific who had "shot prisoners in cold blood, wiped out hospitals, strafed lifeboats, killed or mistreated enemy civilians, finished off the enemy wounded, tossed the dying into a hole with the dead, and in the Pacific boiled the flesh off enemy skulls to make table ornaments for sweethearts, or carved their bones into letter openers. We topped off our saturation bombing and burning of enemy civilians by dropping atomic bombs on two nearly defenseless cities, thereby setting an all-time record for instantaneous mass slaughter."[5]

"As victors," he continued, "we are privileged to try our defeated opponents for their crimes against humanity; but we should be realistic enough to appreciate that if we were on trial for breaking international laws, we should be found guilty on a dozen counts. We fought a dishonorable war, because morality had a low priority in battle. The tougher the fighting, the less room for decency; and in Pacific contests we saw mankind reach the blackest depths of bestiality."

"Not every American soldier," Jones concluded, "or even one per cent of our troops, deliberately committed unwarranted atrocities, and the same might be said for the Germans and Japanese. The exigencies of war necessitated many so-called crimes, and the bulk of the rest could be blamed on the mental distortion which war produced. But we publicized every inhuman act of our opponents and censored any recognition of our own moral frailty in moments of desperation."

——— —— ———

Before Jack Letscher, our battlefield tour guide, dropped me and Ashley off at our hotel, he said he had one more place to show us. Just as the sun began to set along the western horizon, Letscher pulled into a small concrete parking lot facing the ocean. To our left was the Yomitan Village Office and community complex. To our right were several baseball fields, a basketball court, and a running track. Jack said that the area had once been the site of the Yontan Airfield. The name sounded familiar, but I couldn't remember its significance. Jack seemed surprised I hadn't responded to him with more excitement. "This is the same airfield where the B-29 that dropped the atomic bomb on Nagasaki landed."

"Oh, wow!" I said. That reminded me of something my father had told me once. "My father said that my grandfather once made a comment about seeing some big bomber land and knowing that whatever it had been doing was something special. He said there were no fighter planes escorting it and how strange that was."

Letscher then pulled the small stack of papers out from under his seat and leafed through them, licking the tip of his middle finger every few pages. "May 24th," he said, "on order from island command, a patrol from Company C, 193rd Tank Battalion, was sent to Yontan Airfield with the mission of destroying enemy personnel who had made a crash landing on the airstrip." On May 23rd, Letscher explained, 12 Japanese low-flying two-engine bombers took off from an airfield on mainland Japan, near Kyūshū, and flew toward the American-controlled airfield at Yontan. Four encountered mechanical problems and turned back before reaching their intended target. Three more were shot down by American 40-millimeter and 90-millimeter antiaircraft batteries and crashed north of the airfield. Four were intercepted by US night fighters and never got anywhere near the airfield.

The only bomber that remained in the air landed on its belly on Yontan's main runway in the late hours of the night. A young Marine mechanic named Jack Kelly and 17 others from the Marine night fighter squadron were standing on the flight line, getting the F6F Hellcats ready for their nightly missions. They saw the enemy plane skid along the airstrip with its wheels still up, its belly scraping along the pavement, sparks flying. Once the wounded bomber came to a complete stop, Japanese Giretsu commandos armed with rifles, grenades, and satchel charges of TNT rushed out and quickly destroyed nine US planes. Twenty-six other planes were damaged but not destroyed. It was the first and only Japanese airborne assault of the war (not counting Pearl Harbor). After daylight, the bodies of 69 Japanese soldiers were found on or near the airstrip. Ten had been killed at Yontan, and three others were found dead in the plane, evidently killed by antiaircraft fire. The rest had been shot out of the sky and died in fiery wrecks that smoldered and reeked of burned flesh. No prisoners were taken.

Letscher looked up and over to me, then back down to the papers. He scanned some lines before he found what he was looking for: "Okay. Here it is. 'The firing of friendly air force personnel was indiscriminate throughout the night, thus hampering any activity by this unit's patrol. At dawn, a few enemy soldiers who had been hiding at the edge of the field during the night threw several grenades, wounding the S-3, 193rd Tank Battalion.' That's the battalion's operations and training officer. 'These troops were quickly eliminated by small-arms fire from this unit's patrol.'"

"But that wasn't my grandfather's company. He was in Company A," I said.

"That's right," Letscher replied. "So, later that morning, Company A relieved Company C and spent the entire rest of the day patrolling. It doesn't say why Company C had to be relieved. It also says no other enemy soldiers were encountered."

"My father told me a while back," I said, "that after my grandfather's funeral, one of my grandfather's only friends—a Vietnam vet—told my dad that my grandfather had killed a sniper once. Could that have happened after this air raid, during that patrol the next day?"

"It's possible, I suppose," Letscher said. "There's no mention of it in the battalion records here, but that doesn't mean it didn't happen. There are usually discrepancies between records and even between history books."

Then he asked me if I had been able to locate the after-action reports for my grandfather's company. He said those might provide more of the details I was looking for. I told him that I had read the records for April 1945 but that those for May and June had evidently been destroyed in a monsoon after the battle ended. That's what the archivist at the National Archives had told me anyway.

"I can also say," Letscher continued, "that sometimes the men on the ground didn't report certain things up the chain, or the officer preparing the report might have left something out. You have to remember that this was a war of atrocity, and bad things happened all the time—on both sides. Your grandfather, and lots of other men too, I'm sure, were scared and confused and fighting to save themselves and their buddies. Plus, when these records were typed out, the officers writing them probably thought they'd soon have to land on the mainland of Japan. Who knows where their heads were at?"

— — —

When I think about my grandmother, Gladys, and her relationship with my grandfather, I can't help but think about the nature of truth. *What is the truth? What are facts? Isn't the truth simply what we believe based on the facts we have? If so, then don't we need to be open to the idea that what we believe to be true should evolve when new facts come to light?*

From what I've been told, the battering and abuse my grandmother survived were severe and persistent. And it wasn't just physical and emotional. My grandfather was also economically and socially abusive. He didn't let my grandmother have a driver's license or her own money. He was viciously jealous and constantly accused her of running around on him.

What did she think of my grandfather when he came home from the war? Did she notice the changes in him right away, or did it take time for them to develop? What had she expected he was going to be like?

I imagine that my grandmother tried to make sense of it all. She must have tried to understand how my grandfather was feeling. But no matter how hard she tried, she clearly couldn't see things the way he did. There were other boys from town who went to war and came back home and pushed on with their lives. They found girls—or came back to girls—and married and had children and raised families despite whatever was behind them. But not Hod. He went numb and lashed out at others when his numbness wore off. And Gladys didn't know what to do or say about it or how she might help in some way. She felt she did my grandfather no favors by indulging his self-pity. And he resented her for that. It must have been difficult for her to distinguish these moments from the deeper anguish and shame of his war wounds. The children, she had hoped, would soften him. She knew that had happened in her own heart. Her hopes never became reality. My grandfather's drinking intensified, and the violence at home became more frequent.

It was all so sad. Before the war, my grandfather had been a boy on a conference-champion basketball team. He was like other schoolboys in most ways. He had a loyal group of friends. He was a star athlete. He smiled and laughed and talked. In other ways, though, he was different. He drove new cars. His family owned a business that had remained largely untouched by the Great Depression. Anything he ever wanted had been given to him, and he didn't always fully appreciate what he had. He didn't do well in school and dropped out before he graduated. After he had gone to work, his father took him from bar to bar and explained to the owners that his son was a workingman and had his permission to be served. No doubt my grandfather used booze and beer to deal with the emotional upheavals all teenagers experience as they transition from seeking their parents' approval to seeking that of their peers.

When my grandfather returned home from the war, I can imagine that my grandmother was excited at the prospect of who he might have become. She learned soon enough, to her disappointment no doubt, that he was just as flawed as he'd been before he had left. In some ways, he was worse. Even with all the Army and the fighting and the time to mature did to raise him up, my grandfather settled back into his character defects like a dog curling into a round bed. My grandmother soon grew cold. Not exactly hateful, though the distance between her and my grandfather could be felt by anyone paying close enough attention.

Hod needed my grandmother to make life easier for him, and when she refused, he punished her. I see that now. It was easier to lash out at her and abuse her than to deal with the seemingly insurmountable amounts of pain and anger that infected nearly every moment of his life. I imagine he had felt emasculated by her strength and threatened by her intimacy. I don't think it's a stretch to assume he felt intense amounts of shame at his inability to be what others needed him to be.

Perhaps whatever trauma Hod experienced is not to blame for what he ultimately became. Perhaps "it was the war" is too simple of an explanation. What if his wartime experiences had little, if anything, to do with how he treated his family? Maybe the root of his aggression stretches much farther and deeper than the war. If that's true, then perhaps his abusive nature wasn't so much caused by the war as it was magnified by it. Perhaps Patrice is right.

—— —— ——

There's no way I will ever know for sure what happened that day with my grandfather and the prisoner he treated too "softly," according to his platoon leader. All I can do is close my eyes and imagine. This is what I see.

With a handful of rifles and carbines trained on his center mass, the boy stood wearily in the tough grass with his weight mostly on one foot, his back hunched over into the shape of a cashew. When my grandfather barked at the boy to *raise your fucking hands where we can see them*, the boy looked up with a quiet resignation, expecting death, before returning his gaze to my grandfather's mud-caked boots. The boy's hands remained at his side.

The boy might have remained unnoticed if he hadn't reached for the grenade. The Americans' hyperarousal had waned, morphing into an agitation that chewed at whatever self-control they had left. Before my grandfather had found the boy, the Americans had been holding their weapons at a low port in tired arms as they moved their tired eyes from left to right. The shooting from the night before was over, and now it was their job to look for emplacements and hidden stragglers. The weeks-old corpse teeming with maggots the boy had used to cover himself in a ditch near the Yontan Airfield would have probably been more than enough to keep the unshaven and mud-slicked Americans from further investigating the bloated heap of flesh. But then the boy had moved, and my grandfather pounced on his not-dead-yet hand, crushing the boy's metacarpals into the earth.

After they dragged him out from under the rotting body and stripped him to his loincloth, one of the soldiers in the platoon noticed a gangrenous wound on the boy's torso, above his hip and below the bottom of his rib cage. *Looks like he caught a nasty piece of shrapnel*, the soldier said in a soft-spoken voice.

Soon another soldier, a sergeant, waded into the fray. He was rough and tough looking. My grandfather knew him as a tall, slender, and outspoken man who was never at a loss for words. He asked the boy questions much in the same way he berated the junior enlisted. When the boy didn't answer, the sergeant drew his sidearm and poked its barrel into the boy's chest. The boy didn't flinch. The sergeant then raked the tip of the pistol up the boy's sternum and lifted his chin with it so that the boy could watch the words stream out of the sergeant's mouth.

With his head tilted high, the boy blurted out, *I . . . not . . . speaka . . . Engish*. The words shot painfully from his lips like he was spitting out bits of broken glass. Swarms of flies beat out their own tempo as they buzzed in the brief silence that followed.

Bullshit! The sergeant yelled into the boy's face, agitating the flies. This made the boy clam up, which made the sergeant even angrier. He pressed the oily barrel of the pistol between the boy's eyebrows. Seemingly unmoved at first, the boy suddenly crossed his eyes, his heart dropping into his stomach as the sergeant cocked the hammer. Before the trigger could be pulled, the boy found more English words: *School . . . boy. I . . . schoolboy.* He nodded deferentially when the sergeant repeated what he had said.

In a moment of clarity, my grandfather lowered his carbine. *He's just some kid*—a local, he thought. They were all just kids, really. Even the sergeant. They were all scared and wounded, each in his own way, and simply trying to survive this bloody mess. The only difference between my grandfather and this boy was that the boy was not a real soldier. He was an Okinawan conscript forced into service without any training, without a weapon. Little more than cannon fodder. Maybe the grenade wasn't meant for my grandfather and his friends. Maybe it was for the boy himself, to finish the job before the Americans could get their hands on him.

In my mind's eye, I can see my grandfather capturing these images and uploading them somewhere deep in the back of his mind, where they will crowd out happy memories of his wife and baby girl.

Raise your fuckin' rifle! someone snapped at my grandfather. Another soldier prowled back and forth behind the boy, like a loose wolf waiting for caged prey to be released. The man to my grandfather's left was tense and nerve racked. He adjusted his weight and bent his knees slightly. None of them wore packs, just two cans of C-rations in their hip pockets. Changing his stance to a lighter, more alert one, the soldier narrowed his eyes. His rifle was steady and level.

A small bead of sweat rolled into the corner of my grandfather's eye as he tightened his grip on his own weapon. His stomach tingled unpleasantly, almost sickly. His finger hovered gently inside the trigger housing. All it would take to fire would be a gentle squeeze. *Breathe in.*

Breathe out. Hold. Squeeze. It should be a surprise when the recoil slams into your shoulder, he thought to himself.

Aside from the prowling wolf, each of the men tried in the tenseness of the moment to calm themselves and remember their training. It wasn't as automatic as the drill instructors would have liked, but these were tankers, and exceptions had to be made.

The anguished silence was finally broken by a voice of reason. *I'm betting the intel shop will want him. It's not far. We can take him now, get a doc to look at that wound.*

Most of the men in my grandfather's outfit didn't believe in *giving no Jap no chance* anyway, and after fighting them for nearly two months, they believed in it even less than they once had. Instead of thinking through how they might move him to some secure location, they played through various scenarios, each with the same ending. The boy does something—lunges for a weapon, turns to run, pulls out a grenade—for which they can kill him legitimately. The boy probably doesn't understand what they're waiting for. He stares into the distance with acquiescent, pain-dulled eyes.

I say shoot the fucker, my grandfather hears from the soldier prowling behind the boy. *Look at him. Be doin' the poor bastard a favor, you ask me.*

Another soldier chimes in, adding to the chorus: *Let's get this nonsense over with.*

— — —

My goal for this imagined scene was to express my trepidation about my journey to uncover the truth about what my grandfather experienced during the World War II. I wanted to invite you to accompany me down an uncertain path to a destination that I'll never actually reach. I have found that if you fictionalize with grace and openness, showing your vulnerability, you can create intimacy, and the reader will trust you, even though what you're writing is fiction.

The most compelling stories don't simply recount what happened; they also interrogate and engage with what's hidden or unknown. When I began writing about my grandfather and what he experienced overseas, I didn't have much access to his inner life. Not long before my grandfather died, his mother gave him a shoebox full of letters he had sent home during the war, which would probably have been incredibly helpful. Unfortunately, it seems he destroyed them or threw them out, because after he died in August 2000, my father searched all over his one-bedroom shack and found no trace of them. The only military artifacts that remain are a few faded ribbons and a good conduct medal, a wool uniform top, and a dozen or so ochre-tinged photographs. There's one that shows him wearing a garrison cap cocked to the side. He's rubbing his dimpled chin with his left hand. He looks happy, like he had spent the day with good friends and hadn't a care in the world. There are a few of him standing on top of a tank, but those look like they were taken during training maneuvers somewhere. In one, the tank doesn't even have a gun barrel. A black sheet covers the hole where a barrel would normally extend out from the turret.

Then there are a couple of him with a buddy. I don't know his name, though my father thinks he remembers hearing some story about another young man from my grandfather's hometown who was part of the occupation force on Okinawa who ran into my grandfather after the battle ended. His buddy is wearing a suspiciously clean tan service uniform that looks totally out of place. My grandfather, by contrast, is dirt smudged and sweaty looking, wearing dark-green pants tucked into his boots and a white sleeveless shirt. His hair is longer than in the other pictures and waves across his forehead. In three other photographs, his hair still longer and wavy, he's wearing a dark-green top with dark-green pants. The sleeves of his shirt are rolled above his elbows. In the first one, he squats in front of a clay-tiled structure. In the second, he stands with his hands on his hips in front of a thatch-roofed building, and in the third, he's lounging on what appears to be unexploded ordnance as tall as a chair. He looks more like a tourist than an occupying soldier. I don't know who took the pictures.

There are other photographs, too, but they're harder to look at for any length of time. One shows a mass grave of dead bodies from a distance. Another is a close-up of a fallen Japanese soldier. He's lying on his back with his eyes closed. He wears a peaceful smile. His hands rest near his head, as though moments before he'd been standing with his arms raised, silently waiting for death. Whatever thoughts had passed through his mind when the death messenger laid him low seem to have been pleasant enough.

There are also two photographs of Japanese soldiers just after they surrendered. The last two show a prisoner of war camp. The first is of the camp's main gate. About 15 young Japanese men in baggy, mucky uniforms are marching through it, away from the photographer. None of their faces are visible. The other photograph shows 75 or so docile and pathetic-looking Japanese and Okinawan men, most stripped down to their loincloths, standing nuts to butts behind razor wire as tall as a man. An American military policeman with a Thompson submachine gun stands guard in the foreground.

I have tried on several occasions to enter the moments of these photos, imagining their context, what might have happened outside the frame in the moments before or after the shutter clicked. I took what I knew about my grandfather and what I could imagine of the younger version of him, and I created a scene that breathes life into the moments captured by the camera. I felt comfortable doing this because I wasn't inventing details to "improve on" the facts; rather, I was actively and transparently engaging with questions of truth and identity. *Who were these people?* I wondered.

If we censor ourselves by refusing to allow speculation and imagination into memoir, then we're closing a door on an important aspect of our lives—the time we all spend daydreaming and thinking about the past and future. I believe that if our goal is to understand our own stories and to use them to connect with others—and not just to document what happened—then speculating or imagining our way into our material is crucial to the endeavor.

If this technique interests you, I would suggest starting in one of three places. First, you could try writing the dialogue of a conversation you always wanted to have but never had. Second, you could put one of the characters in your story on an imaginary soapbox and allow them to speak through your words about themselves or about a topic of interest to you. Last, if you've already tried to write your story but have gotten stuck because your memory is hazy, or because you didn't witness an important event or development, write the scene as you think it unfolded. As you do this, make it clear to readers that you are imagining and tell them why you need to do this.

— — —

I'm sympathetic to the struggle some of you will have when it comes to recording your memories. When details are fuzzy and speculations too numerous, it can be hard to find the right balance. There are blurry lines between what happened, how we remember what happened, and how we'd prefer to remember it. If you find yourself struggling with the details of your story, ask yourself whether the detail is all that important. If it isn't, leave it out or tell the reader you cannot remember exactly what happened by saying, "I could have been . . ." or "I don't remember exactly, but . . ." or "It's possible that . . ." or the like. If the detail does matter, ask yourself whether it's worth the emotional effort to retrieve it and make a plan to take care of yourself as you fill in the gaps.

I also recommend writing down your memories without input from others. This will ensure your stories are truly your own. Once you have your memories recorded, try researching your story's key events. What was the weather like that day? What songs were most popular? What were the leading news stories? Then find a copy of a newspaper issued that day. Listen to the popular music again. If the sun was shining that day, go out on a sunny day to see if doing so triggers anything for you. Pay attention to any sensations you feel in your body, and record those as well. A visceral sensation is muscle memory in action.

The stories we tell ourselves can sometimes feel like clothes we need to try on in the fitting room before taking them home. Some don't fit as well as we'd hoped. Others are outrageous and can't be pulled off. We put them on, stare into the mirror, and try to imagine ourselves in another place at another time. If they don't quite fit or suit our figure, we can take them off and try on some other look, some other style.

There's a beauty in the search. And there's triumph in the telling—as long as you're honest with your reader.

References

1. Dorothy Parker, "Who Is That Man?," *Vogue*, July 1944, 67. Parker's article was reproduced in condensed form in *Reader's Digest* under the title "Discussional Springboard." Readers were encouraged to respond to Parker's article, and some of the responses were printed in an article titled "But Will He Return a Stranger?," *Reader's Digest*, July 1944.

2. J. C. Furnan, "Meet Ed Savickas," *Ladies' Home Journal* 62 (February 1945): 141–44. See also Doris Weatherford, *American Women during World War II: An Encyclopedia* (New York: Taylor and Francis, 2009), 494.

3. Thomas Childers, *Soldier from the War Returning: The Greatest Generation's Troubled Homecoming from World War II* (New York: Houghton Mifflin Harcourt, 2009), 93.

4. Irene Stokes Culman, "Now Stick with Him," *Good Housekeeping*, May 1945, 17.

5. Edgar L. Jones, "One War Is Enough," *Atlantic Monthly*, February 1946, https://www.theatlantic.com/past/docs/unbound/bookauth/battle/jones.htm.

9

Telling Your Story to Build Connection and Understanding

Back when I was still teaching a writing seminar to student veterans at the University of Wisconsin–Stevens Point, I'd wake long before the sun came up and brew a pot of coffee before heading downstairs to my dimly lit office. The house I lived in then was built in 1871, when insulating a basement wasn't much of a priority. In the wintertime, it was especially cold down there, but I didn't mind it. My work had a way of warming me until the coffee was done. To begin, I would sit down at my desk—a castoff I'd found in the university surplus store—and open my laptop.

On one particularly cold morning, I opened the essay draft that Mike had sent me the week before and read it without typing or trying to fix anything. I made that a habit after the student I told you about in the introduction had such a traumatizing reaction to his essay. By forcing myself to take in the whole piece, without trying to fix it right away, I can better gauge whether it's accomplishing what the writer wants—or not.

I didn't know much about Mike Goranson when I started working with him on his essay. All I knew was that he was captain of the Chicago chapter of Team Red, White & Blue (Team RWB is a nonprofit that

helps veterans adjust to civilian life) and that he was finally ready—
after more than a decade—to tell his story. Before my first cup of coffee that morning, I'd already learned quite a bit more about Mike. In
"Alive Day" he'd written about the day he almost died in Iraq and the
difficulties he later faced when he got home.

It was November 29, 2004, and Mike was a Marine deployed to Ra-
madi. The rest of his unit was conducting a door-to-door patrol while
he and another Marine guarded a T-intersection outside. An insurgent
popped out from behind a building and fired off a burst from his AK-
47. One of the rounds ricocheted off Mike's truck and struck him in the
ankle, just above the top of his boot. The round burst through the back
of his leg, and Mike began bleeding uncontrollably.

Before he bled out, he was able to radio in that he needed to be evac-
uated. Not long after, another truck came to Mike's rescue. He doesn't
remember much from the rest of that day, except the corpsman helping him into the truck and hearing mortars landing near the field hospital as the anesthesia kicked in before the first of many surgeries.

After the field surgeons in Iraq were able to stop his bleeding, Mike
was flown to an American military hospital in Germany for more surgery. From there, he was sent to Walter Reed in Washington, DC,
where the doctors told him there was a chance he was going to lose his
foot. Fortunately, it never came to that, though he did sustain perma-
nent tibial nerve damage. Once he was healed enough to head home to
Illinois, he was given a hero's welcome, complete with a call from the
mayor.

All was going relatively well for Mike and his recovery until he flew
to San Diego to welcome back the rest of his unit from their deployment. It was then that a buddy told him that the other Marine he'd
been with the day he'd been hit had told everyone in the unit that Mike
had given up on the fight after he was shot, that he had quit.

When I came back to my desk after finishing that first cup of coffee,
I wasn't sure if I could read Mike's essay again. It seemed he still had
lots of processing to do. His language and tone were defensive, and I
had the overwhelming sense that he was searching more for absolution

than for understanding. He wanted me, the reader, to believe him—that he hadn't quit, that no one knows how they're going to react when they get shot, and that he had done the best he could. My stomach ached in anxiety over what I could possibly say to help him with his story.

Mike's first draft seemed to be his first attempt at answering the ultimate question: *Why did this happen to me?* Questions like this, questions that begin with *why*, assume an architectural order to the universe I don't believe actually exists. When we ask *why*, what we're really saying is that we want this universal order revealed so that we might feel like we're standing on solid ground. When the order remains hidden, as Mike seemed to have concluded, we are left believing that either we are incapable of finding it or that the universe is built on shifting sand.

—— —— ——

I met Mike for the first time at a Panera in downtown Chicago. I arrived at the restaurant before Mike did, hoping that if I got there first, maybe it would signal to him that I took the meeting seriously and that I wasn't just some guy dropping in to hand out life and writing advice like prescription meds at the VA.

I had seen pictures of Mike on Facebook, so I knew what he looked like: dark, short hair; baby face unmarred by a razor; kind eyes; and a sheepish grin. When he arrived, I was surprised by how tall he was. I'm six feet four inches and played defensive line on my college football team, but Mike towered over me.

We shook hands, and I introduced myself. I could tell by the way he was looking at me—sizing me up, really—and by the way he was standing, at a diagonal to me, that he was apprehensive. He knew I had read his story, but I hadn't given him feedback yet. I wanted to talk with him about my first reactions, rather than send them in an email. It was like a first date. I couldn't help but wonder what he was thinking, and he seemed to be aching to know what I was thinking.

We turned to face the menu board and Mike blurted out, "So, where'd you serve?"

I hate that question. I get it all the time. "I'm actually not a veteran," I said. "I work with them, help them tell their stories." I could tell he was disappointed. He nodded his head and looked away, as if to say, *Great, this fuckin' guy.* He didn't say another word, except to order his lunch, until we sat down to eat.

As Mike took the first big bite of his sandwich, I cut straight to the chase: "Take me back to that day," I told him.

"Nobody really knows how they're going to react when they get hit," he said after swallowing his first bite. He then told me that after he got hit, he dropped his machine gun in the dirt and scrambled for cover. He made a point of saying that even though he didn't have his big gun, he still had his sidearm. He said he would have died if he hadn't dropped the big gun and called in his injury. He was leaning forward, elbows on the table that separated us. It seemed to me that he had rehearsed the events in his mind over and over again but had not yet explored either his emotions or the meaning of his story. He didn't look away or hang his head as he talked. I could feel how badly he wanted me to believe him.

He told me how he felt his heart drop when he heard what some of the other guys had said about thinking he'd quit. "And worst of all," he continued, "the guy who said that shit died in a motorcycle crash a couple of days later, so I never even got a chance to confront him about what he said."

Only then did I understand where all the defensiveness was coming from. Mike was still hurting, more than 10 years later. He didn't want his fellow Marines—anyone, really—to think he was a quitter. He was a good Marine. He had served honorably. He knew that, but it still hurt to think there were people who thought differently.

The problem with the first draft of Mike's essay was that it was a confession. I don't mean that he did something wrong and felt the need to be forgiven. It's more complicated than that. He knew he had done the best he could, but the other guys in his unit didn't believe that. He told his story not to get me to better understand him but rather to get me to take his side and to believe that he was the person he thought he was. Instead of ripping open his shirt and showing me his prover-bial scars, he simply spilled his guts, like a drunk vomiting in the gut-ter after a long night of shots. The experience may have been cathar-tic for Mike, but it did nothing to help me connect with him.

In all honesty, Mike's essay made me feel bad for him, even pity him. And that's not what Mike was looking for. He was in a good place when we met for the first time, and he wanted to tell his story so others could know who he was, what he had been through, and why he does what he does now.

I had so many questions for him. I barely ate my own food. Mike, to his credit, answered truthfully, like one friend confiding in another. As he talked, I jotted down his answers in a small notebook. The more he talked, the more he seemed to decompress. His shoulders, which had been pulled up to his ears most of the time we were together, be-gan to relax. He laughed and smiled more. It no longer seemed to matter that I had never had an experience similar to his.

When we were finished, I ripped out the sheets of paper with my notes and gave them to him. "This is your story," I told him. "No one else's. Not your friend's. Not anyone's. Just yours. Tell the reader what *you* went through and how *you* felt. Don't try to put words in others' mouths or defend yourself against what they *might* say. Don't make ex-cuses or try to defend yourself. Confide in the reader, and the reader will connect with you on a level you can't even believe."

I believe that good storytellers are generous, even to unsympathetic and unredeemable characters. If we, as writers, avoid self-pity, whin-ing, and the need for vengeance, if we are honest about our own sins and shortcomings, our readers will see our humanity. This under-standing of the private self's story and its place in a greater context is crucial for one writer's trauma to transcend personal significance and enter the realm of public significance. Plus, I'll guarantee that if you portray the people in your story as three-dimensional, focusing on both the negative and the positive aspects of who they are, their true nature will show through regardless, and you can avoid coming across as biased.

My goal for Mike—the reason I read his story, met with him, and told him how it made me feel—was to convince him that there was a way he could tell his story so that it would provide space for readers to furnish their own knowledge where his breaks down, to apply the ideas in his writing to their own opinions and purposes.

After Team RWB published Mike's revised essay on its blog, I shared a link to it on Facebook. A good friend of mine—who's also a civilian— sent me a message to tell me how much she connected with Mike's story. "I've never been in combat or anything," she wrote, "but I know exactly what it feels like to think I've let someone down." My friend connected with Mike's story because it wasn't really about war. It was about simply being human, about feeling like a failure, and about doing the best you can anyway.

Confessing and Confiding

About a year after Mike's story was published, I was teaching a story-telling workshop at a retreat center on an island off the coast of Seattle. By that point in my teaching career, I had converted my experience working with Mike into a short lecture on how to connect with readers and create understanding with stories of trauma. The PowerPoint slide I created to go along with the lecture had two columns. The column on the left was labeled "Confession," and the column on the right was labeled "Confidence." Under each label, I listed several characteristics of stories that could be considered confessional or confidential, respectively. My goal was to show how Mike's story had evolved from a confession where he felt he had to "spill his guts" to a confidence in which he was able to articulate what happened to him, how it made him feel, and what he learned from the experience.

Confessional stories, I told the group of military veterans and their family members, were seemingly addressed to God, a court, the public, or a person who may have been wronged—something or someone who has power over you. Confessionals can read like they are, and oftentimes feel, coerced—like the writer isn't ready to share. I can usually tell when this is the case because the writer is overly occupied with narration and content: *this happened, and then this happened, and then this happened.*

Confessional stories are, by definition, emotionally charged and usually show only one side of the story, which can have an intense and disruptive effect on a reader who doesn't know the writer and therefore cannot condemn or forgive. Think about what I told you about the first draft of Mike's story. He felt ashamed of what his friend had told the rest of his platoon. What response would he have had if I had told him he was forgiven? Or if I condemned him? But I have no skin in that game; whatever I think about what he did is immaterial. If I were his priest, that would be a different matter altogether. But I'm not a priest.

Confessional stories, moreover, tend to lack perspective and portray characters as one-dimensional. Perhaps most importantly, this type of story, I've found, tends to hide from the hard truths, and it is the hard truths that readers tend to connect with most.

What I call confidential stories—think *confiding* in a friend—on the other hand are purposefully addressed to a reader who can chide, laugh, or weep but who has no authority to condemn or forgive the writer. Confidential stories help build relationships by affording writers, not an opportunity to spill their guts, but rather to roll up their sleeves and expose their scars to the light of day.

Confidential stories are always volunteered, even though they can be as emotional as confessional stories. Because the goal of confidential stories is to build connection, they must be focused more on showing all sides of the story, portraying characters as three-dimensional, and shedding light on hard truths. Whereas confessional stories are all about content, confidential stories are about creating and furthering relationships and understanding.

I was proud of my insights, having thought critically about what Mike needed to ensure that his story would lead to connection and understanding. I thought I had figured out an ingenious way to help my students avoid scaring their readers away with their confessional stories of trauma.

And then I met a young woman who jolted me out of my false sense of security. Even now, years later, I can see her face in my mind's eye. I can see her eyes, dry at first, then welling with tears of anger. I can see her sitting, bolt upright, on a brown leather couch, her back straight as an arrow. I can see her ready to burst at the word *confessional*, shocked that I would dare suggest it was the writer's job to bring comfort to the reader. I can see her flanked on both sides by women who have also begun to cry.

Before that lecture, I did not know that woman well. We had spent only a couple of days together at the retreat center. She was my student, and I was her teacher, and there were two dozen other students who needed my attention. I cannot recall if we'd had even a single one-on-one interaction before that lecture. My memory tells me we did not.

By that point in the storytelling workshop, we had already talked about post-traumatic growth and the ways in which people can transform in the face of adversity. She and the rest of the students had inventoried the positive ways they had changed as a result of the trauma they experienced. We talked about scene building and the essentials of storytelling and how immersive details can bring the reader fully into the story.

The most engaging discussion we'd had as a class centered on starting with one true thing, like Hemingway had done, and on uncovering the object of desire—that thing you desire above all else—and on how sometimes getting closer to the thing you want leads you farther way from what you really need. From what I could tell, this woman and the rest of the students understood the point of these exercises and were beginning to see the ways in which truly impactful stories can be crafted.

When she raised her hand to speak, I didn't know what to expect. I almost never do. Most of the time, students in my workshops ask clarifying questions that I can easily answer by expanding on a point or by sharing one of the many instructional anecdotes I've collected over the years. I've learned how to think quickly on my feet and to redirect and reframe comments that steer the class off course or disrupt the flow of my lesson.

Before I could call on her, she stood and addressed the rest of the group as much as she was addressing me. She said that since the abuse began, she had not felt empowered to speak her truth. She hid the results of the abuse and the emotions she couldn't seem to control because the people in her life who were supposed to take care of her refused to believe the truth. Rather than comfort her, they expected her to make others feel comfortable. Her only option, she said, was to turn off the tears, push down any inconvenient emotions, and soldier on.

I do not know the details of her trauma. And even if I did, they're not mine to share. What I do know is that the idea of using her story to bring comfort to her readers was such an offensive proposition that she stood and spoke her truth to me and to everyone else who was there that day.

I wish I could say that I responded to her appropriately. I fear I did not. When her story veered into a dismissal of my lesson on confession and confidence, I wanted to stop her before she could finish. I wanted to defend myself, to explain that I wasn't saying what she thought I was saying. I wanted her to understand my message: that testifying to trauma or abuse and detailing the worst days of our lives was not what we were there to do. I wanted to reiterate that we were talking about using our stories of survival and growth to build connection and understanding, not to turn our readers off. But I was afraid to stop her. So I stood silent.

When she told her parents what had happened, she said, they did not want to believe her. Nothing could change their minds. It seems that was the deepest cut of all.

I became a teacher because I'm driven by a need to help others navigate their emotional landscapes with more confidence. I know what it feels like to live inside a story that prevents you from living the life you desire. After years of navigating my own uncharted landscapes, I had convinced myself that I had the map and a compass and a flashlight, too, and that what I had learned could help people. When this woman said what she said, and as the two women next to her hugged her and handed her tissues, I knew I had to say *something*.

All I could muster was that I had not explained my point clearly enough. I felt confused. And then horrified. That afternoon was the first time in my teaching career that someone had admonished me for something I thought I had said so deftly; I couldn't call up the compassionate and empathetic response I wish I could have.

Looking around the room as the seconds of utter silence ticked by in my head, I saw the horror on some of the students' faces. Or was that pity? Was it pity for her? Or for me? Were they embarrassed for me? It was so hard for me to tell. My horror quickly exploded into shame. A fire raged through a canyon choked with tinder, my hot heart burning. I could sense by so many others' open mouths and shocked stares that they could feel what I was feeling. I got the sense that they too wanted that moment to end, that they wanted someone to put out the fire.

— — —

It took a long time for me to be honest with myself about that day. She was not to blame for how I felt inside. I didn't listen to what she said. Instead, I heard her say that I was part of the problem—that my offering was not a solution. Time and reflection and conversation with others who teach writing have helped me realize that in overwrought workshop moments, when a misunderstanding arises, I can maintain a connection with my students, convey my message, and reestablish trust that may have been shaken.

I wish she were willing to speak with me again, but she is not. I can't say I blame her. I do want her to know—maybe she'll read this someday—that I had no intention of retraumatizing her or anyone else. I also want her to know that if I could go back in time to that day, to that moment, I would tell myself to listen and to say how proud I am that she had the courage to share. I would let her know how impressed I was that she never made peace with mediocrity. Whatever bitterness she may have harbored didn't stop her from striving for more, from being more.

It's important that you and every other writer remind yourself that if there ever comes a time when someone struggles to believe what you say, you should understand that the root cause of such incredulity does not testify to your inferiority but rather to their fear. Many people find it hard to act on what they know to be true. To act is to be committed, and to be committed is to risk loss. And I would say—and I hope I wouldn't be out of line—that there is no reason for you to make others feel comfortable at your own expense.

There's one more thing I want to say: Tell your story. Tell it with your whole self, whether it brings comfort to others or not. Tell it as though it is all that has ever mattered. I cannot stress enough how much it matters that you do this. Stories, after all, are what save us.

Afterword

ANGELA RICKETTS
Author of *No Man's War*

M y teenagers introduced me to The 1975, an angsty, irreverent but "woke" pop band. Not long ago, I caught the lyrics to one of the band's songs, a mantra that stuck with me because of its blatant, simplified explanation for navigating trauma or escaping the drowning of one horrible day: "If you can't survive, just try." Read that simple refrain again. And then again.

The choice to delve into Dave Chrisinger's guide to writing about trauma is a big step in the right direction. Writing about personal hells takes courage, self-awareness, and examination. The word *trauma* can appear to be tired—like the word *resilient*. Both have become buzzwords used ad nauseam in the context of dealing with the inevitable shitstorms of life. Because our vernacular is sorely lacking adequate synonyms for the word *trauma*, *shitstorm* and *personal horror* have become my own favorites. Especially given that as I write these words, we are, as a global community, currently waist deep in an unprecedented pandemic. Let's not allow the potency behind the word *trauma* to be reduced to monotonous white noise.

Let's face it; life is a series of private storms or commonly shared but differently experienced storms. Why do we feel the most compelled to write about our awful moments, with intermittent happy stuff sprinkled in? And why does human nature fuel us with the need to look for happy endings? Maybe the pressure to find that happy ending perpetuates another level of trauma all its own.

There is value in finding the words to express trauma; it's absolutely transformative. But here's the thing about expressing our personal horrors—well, two things. The first thing: you have to be ready. The second thing: you'll never be ready. You can't write trauma away, but writing can be an effective tool for alleviating the burden of trauma and serving as a vehicle of comprehension. Writing into the trauma gives clarity and sometimes can even give the trauma an identity of its own.

One disclaimer before I dig into this afterword about my own experience with trauma writing: I can't promise that I won't throw a bunch of cringe-worthy clichés into the air just to see how many I can dodge or catch. The thing about clichés is that they're usually based in fact. Facts are universal, objective, yet elusive. Facts are also subjective and personal. But the truth in clichés will get you every time.

I call bullshit on the notion that trauma builds character or resilience. Trauma doesn't result in resilience. It hardens us. It erodes and erases us. Trauma robs us of the ability to be still—to be quiet. I used to be funny. I used to have an ironclad memory. I used to speak in complete sentences. I used to avoid passive voice like the plague. My personal avalanche of trauma has stolen the person I used to be.

Trauma is not an event. The easiest way to deal with trauma is to put it in a box (as I did with a trauma I endured as a newlywed in my early twenties, which I reluctantly included in my 2014 memoir). Writing about trauma means opening that sealed box, taking the trauma out, making eye contact, and holding it. It's almost like having your arm trapped and knowing the only path to survival is to chew it off. You know you need to get it over with, but you also know it's gonna hurt like hell. Trauma doesn't care how long you procrastinate. It waits patiently with no place else to be. Writing your trauma gives it an identity of its own, and that alone offers a powerful release. You can't escape trauma, but you can write it out of the path you need to follow to move forward. Writing allows you to see the trauma for what it is, a thing that exists apart from you and also in you. It's possible that, by writing, you will learn to coexist with your shitstorm like a conjoined twin who can't be avoided.

We can study trauma, read about it, and think we understand the horrors others live through; yet no matter how much you've learned secondhand, when it happens to you, it feels like it's the first time it has ever happened to someone in the history of humankind. Any attempt to measure traumatic events against other traumatic events or especially other people's traumas is simplistic. Each trauma is singular and specific.

About a year before an unfathomable trauma unleashed itself on my family's world, my memoir about my lifetime inside the insular subculture of the infantry community was published to a flurry of buzz, media, and brouhaha. That experience was titillating, and my skin thickened quickly. The quest for how to end my memoir had been agony for me. While writing a memoir, the elusive arrival at a happy ending becomes a writer's albatross. I ended that book at the wedding of one of my most beloved characters. The wedding site was a picturesque lake on a perfect summer day. It was one step shy of a contrived walk into the sunset. The truth is that my beloved character's new marriage didn't stick, and he'd landed in divorce purgatory before my book came out. I could have changed the ending, but I didn't. No one wants to read a story with a miserable ending.

We live in a culture that promises a happy ending to a story. Not to be a bummer, but here's a little secret: happy endings don't exist. In fact, those two words are in complete contradiction with each other. Happy and ending. Tracy Letts wrote, "If we knew the future, we'd never get out of bed." Memoirs by definition are a snapshot of a longer life. That snapshot has to be worked into a story with a beginning, a middle, and . . . a satisfying conclusion. There must be a struggle, a story arc, and a resolution, even in nonfiction. We can pretend to tie things up in a neat bow, but that bow will eventually unravel.

All that aside, after my memoir came out, I thought I'd skate through the rest of whatever life tossed into my path. The worst just had to be over. As far as I was concerned, the most tumultuous yet beautiful time of my life was behind me. Naively, I craved a boring ending.

— — —

A memoir is an interpretation of a memory, and memories are tricky. If I'd written my memoir relying solely on my memory, it would have brimmed with inaccuracies and untruths. As I painstakingly scoured decades' worth of detailed journals for material, I realized that the notes I'd made from memory alone were often incorrect. I'm not sure why memories are often incorrect. Maybe the brain rewrites personal history as a subconscious survival mechanism. Our memories alone, especially traumatic memories, are never a reliable source. In the end, I was proud of the unflinching and raw stories I told. Many people were perturbed by what I'd written, and some criticized me, but no one ever called me a liar. I can live with that.

My own overall story was just beginning where my book had left off, but I didn't know that when my book came out. For many years I used my most traumatic event from my early twenties as fuel to survive other shitstorms that were far less shitty by comparison. Who knows how many readers walked away with that impression, but there it was: me spelling it out. The trauma I didn't want to include at all wormed its way into becoming the moral of that story. One traumatic event represented my inner tenacity for two decades of war chaos to follow.

I find the very word *memoir* to be gross, entitled, and narcissistic sounding. When asked what I write, my preferred answer is nonfiction. My story felt socially and historically relevant, yet I was never comfortable with the pretentiousness of the word *memoir*. If pressed, I say it was a book about my time as a war wife, but that sums it up too neatly. I was never good at the elevator pitch. Memoir writing is tricky because you don't want it to seem like it's all about you, but a memoir is all about you and your place in one picture or a few in a lifetime photo album. The act of memoir writing is an intimate purge. It's been five years since my *memoir*, and I don't even know that main character anymore. That person who *was* a version of myself, a flawed, struggling character who acted as both the protagonist and antagonist. Readers see me as a character, the caricature of myself I chose to portray in that singular moment and role. That self-made depiction of myself is out there, forever, for better or worse. Regardless of the fresh storms of hell that have unleashed and changed me as a person, those published words give permission for others to forever see me as the character I painted.

But life moves on. Life rolls us over when we least expect it.

— — —

It's been nearly four years since my healthy, thriving, athletic, wicked-funny, conscientious 17-year-old son, Jack, was diagnosed with a rare and possibly terminal brain tumor. I am stuck in the details of that day four years ago. I was sitting in our living room and watching a movie with my kids. I can still hear the phone ring. I can remember thinking, *huh, yesterday they said to expect a call next week with the hospital's test results.* I'd paused the after-school, snowy-day movie and handed my youngest daughter the bowl of popcorn we'd been sharing. Our attempt to pretend everything was normal had been a weak struggle. I still have the little half piece of paper I'd used to scribble down the unfamiliar words as quickly as the doctor had spoken them. Now, when I look at that piece of paper, I find it perversely quaint that I misspelled the part of my 17-year-old son's brain where they had found a tumor.

The doctor paused often as he spoke and asked me if I understood what he'd said. I scrawled, "one in a mill." I had started to use numerals, but in my confusion I couldn't make sense of how many zeros I needed. The doctor gave me a website to go to for more information. "Hope for HH." The H in the acronym stood for Hope. *Wait, what?* This situation requires hope? It's been almost four years, and I can still see myself hanging up the phone, then unpausing *The Help*. We'd been watching the scene right at the end where Miss Hilly accuses Aibileen of stealing silver, and then Aibileen asks Miss Hilly, "Aren't you tired?" In retrospect, I see the painful irony of that scene. Yes, Aibileen. I am tired, and too old for this shit . . . this new storm of shit.

Trauma in the first half of a lifetime builds character and wisdom. In the second half of life, it feels different. For me, it feels corrosive. Kind of like that old adage that says we spend the first half of our lives acquiring material stuff and the second half of life ridding ourselves of that stuff. Trauma in the second half of life takes a steeper toll. When I was in my twenties and thirties, I'd read Mary Higgins Clark novels and emulated Martha Stewart, or tried to. I was eager, prepared, and ahead of all situations. Even the shitshows.

My memory of the rest of that day Jack's neurosurgeon called isn't as clear. I remember that none of it felt real. I don't think I cried until the next day, and then I cried for weeks and months. I still cry today.

I wish someone in those early weeks had told me to take care of myself and my two younger daughters. Maybe they did tell me that, and I just don't remember. That's the thing about trauma. Your brain maxes out at a certain point, and words begin to sound like Charlie Brown's teacher.

I wish a lot of things when I look back to the spring of 2016. I wish I had known that our family wasn't experiencing an acute event but rather entering a chronic and relentless new way of life, one where crisis and chaos dictated our new normal. I wish I had known the irreversible change this would bring for my sweet daughters. I wish I would have paid attention to the possible outcomes and what Jack's life might look like if he survived. Back then the only word we heard was *survival*. I question whether I would have paid attention to Jack's wishes if I could go back. I wish, even now, that I knew how to move forward. That's another thing about trauma. There's an awful lot of wishing you could go back and handle it differently or avoid it altogether. Maybe I wish I hadn't been able to grasp the magnitude of the suck. That was a fresh suck that couldn't be withstood.

Three years and two months after that day I'd scribbled notes on that piece of scrap paper, I was sitting in the car on a textbook-perfect spring day, with my sunroof open despite the darkness I felt inside, and talking on the phone with Dave Chrisinger. He asked me to write this afterword. Dave knew that Jack had struggled since his tumor diagnosis, but as I explained that Jack was hospitalized and fighting for his life again, I began to cry. Maybe even sob. But I agreed to write this afterword for his book, and I knew it would hurt to see the words in black and white. Proof that happy endings are fairy tales. Ultimately, I suppose, that's the goal: acceptance of what is real and messy but somehow retains a measure of beauty.

All of this seems incredibly bleak, and maybe it is, but we have no choice but to endure. I like to think of resilience as a form of wisdom. It makes me loathe the word a little less to think that I haven't just weathered a storm but have gained wisdom along the way. Joni Mitchell summed it up best with her lyrics: "Something's lost, but something's gained/In living every day." And Stevie Nicks wonders if she can handle the seasons of her life, and so do I.

So don't bother trying to rid yourself of trauma altogether. Forget about happy endings. You will lose. Escaping trauma isn't unlike trying to swim out of a riptide. The best you can do is swim parallel to the riptide, which goes against every natural instinct to fight the undercurrent to escape. Riptides at least allow a chance of escape and a happy ending. That's where riptides and trauma part ways. Swim with the trauma and maybe you'll see happier days with the wisdom that everything, including happiness and trauma, is temporary.

— — —

Angela Ricketts's first memoir, No Man's War: Irreverent Confessions of an Infantry Wife, was critically lauded and featured on NPR's Fresh Air. Angela has appeared on MSNBC and CNN. She is a reluctant but periodic guest on Fox News. She is a graduate of Indiana University and holds a master's degree in social psychology. She has traveled the country advocating for veteran and military family issues, including speaking at the Los Angeles Times Festival of Books. Her childhood as an army brat and 26 years as an army wife have allowed her to live around the world. After 38 moves, she has now settled permanently with her husband and family of three children in Bloomington, Indiana. In addition to consulting for various mental health organizations, Angela is currently hard at work on a second memoir.

Transformation Inventory

Mark the appropriate box beside each possible area of growth to indicate the degree to which you transformed because of your experience(s):

- 1 = I transformed to a small degree or not at all.
- 2 = I transformed to a moderate degree.
- 3 = I transformed to a great degree.

Possible Areas of Transformation	1	2	3
My priorities about what is important in life have changed.			
I better appreciate the value of my own life.			
I developed new interests.			
I am self-reliant.			
I have a stronger religious or spiritual faith.			
I can count on people in times of trouble.			
I established a new path for my life.			
I have a sense of closeness with others.			
I am more willing to express my emotions.			
I can handle difficulties.			
I can now do better things with my life.			
I can accept the way things work out.			
I have new opportunities that I may not have had otherwise.			
I have more compassion for others.			
I put more effort into my relationships.			
I am better able to change things that need to be changed.			
I am stronger than I thought I was.			
I accept needing others.			

"I believe . . ."

Once you have finished filling out the Transformation Inventory, pick one to three of the areas you marked as ones of significant change.

Step 1. For at least one of these areas of change, complete the sentences started below to express how you believe you changed as a result of your experience.

I believe that _____

_____

_____

I also believe that _____

_____

_____

In addition, I believe that _____

_____

_____

Step 2. Answer the question "How so?" (How did you come to believe these things about your experience?)

_____

_____

_____

_____

_____

_____

_____

_____

Step 3. Answer the question "Why?" (Why did you change what you believed about your experience?)

_____

_____

_____

_____

_____

_____

_____

_____

Your Object of Desire

Step 1. Determine what it is that you wanted in the story you're telling and finish the sentences below.

I wanted _____

_____

_____

_____

I also wanted _____

_____

_____

_____

_____

Step 2. Finish the sentences below by describing what you did to get what you wanted.

To get what I wanted, I _____

_____

_____

_____

_____

I then _____

_____

_____

_____

_____

Step 3. Figure out what your obstacle was and what you did to overcome it.
Finish the sentences below.

Before I could get what I wanted, _____

_____

_____

_____

_____

So I _____

_____

_____

_____

_____

Five Essentials of Storytelling

First Essential. Inciting event: What happened that knocked you out of your routine or upset the balance of your life?

_____

_____

_____

_____

_____

Second Essential. Progressive complications: What conflicts did you encounter in trying to get what you wanted?

_____

_____

_____

_____

_____

Third Essential. Crisis: What choices did you have when you realized you must make a decision?

_____

_____

_____

_____

_____

_____

Fourth Essential. Climax: What did you do when you made your decision?

_____

_____

_____

_____

_____

Fifth Essential. Resolution: What resulted from the decision you made?

_____

_____

_____

_____

_____

_____

Starting with One True Thing

Step 1. Write three sentences that could be good first lines for your story.

1. _____

   _____

   _____

   _____

   _____

2. _____

   _____

   _____

   _____

   _____

3. _____

   _____

   _____

   _____

   _____

Step 2. Read your three sentences out loud, and ask yourself these questions about them:

- Which of the sentences resonates the most with me?
- Which is the most interesting?
- What questions would I have after hearing each sentence if I didn't know the rest of the story?

Articles and Essays on the Craft of Memoir and Writing about Trauma

Ackerman, Angela. "Writing about Pain without Putting Your Readers in Agony." Writers Helping Writers, February 9, 2017. http://writershelping writers.net/2017/02/how-to-accurately-write-about-your-characters-pain/.

Appleton Pine, Sarah. "The Structure of Trauma." *Ploughshares* (blog), March 1, 2019. http://blog.pshares.org/index.php/the-structure-of -trauma/.

Bereola, Abigail. "A Reckoning Is Different than a Tell-All: An Interview with Kiese Laymon." *Paris Review* (blog), October 18, 2018. https://www .theparisreview.org/blog/2018/10/18/a-reckoning-is-different-than-a-tell -all-an-interview-with-kiese-laymon/.

Chee, Alexander. "Annie Dillard and the Writing Life." *Morning News*, October 16, 2009. https://themorningnews.org/article/annie-dillard-and -the-writing-life.

Chung, Nicole. "Amy Tan on Writing and the Secrets of Her Past." Shonda- land, October 16, 2017. https://www.shondaland.com/inspire/books /a12919749/amy-tan-interview/.

Cooper, Bernard. "Marketing Memory." LA Weekly, February 24, 1999. https://www.laweekly.com/marketing-memory/.

Jerkins, Morgan. "But What Will Your Parents Think?" *Longreads*, May 2018. https://longreads.com/2018/05/10/but-what-will-your-parents -think/.

Madden, T Kira. "Against Catharsis: Writing Is Not Therapy." Lit *Hub*, March 22, 2019. https://lithub.com/against-catharsis-writing-is-not -therapy/.

Reid, Ruthanne. "Show, Don't Tell: How to Write the Stages of Grief." *Write Practice*, n.d. http://thewritepractice.com/writing-grief/.

Rowbottom, Allie. "Writing Truthfully about My Father: An Act of Resistance, an Act of Love." *Salon*, July 27, 2018. https://www.salon.com/2018/07/27 /writing-truthfully-about-my-father-an-act-of-resistance-an-act-of-love.

Sayrafiezadeh, Said. "How to Write about Trauma." *New York Times*, August 14, 2016. https://www.nytimes.com/2016/08/14/opinion/sunday/how-to-write-about-trauma.html.

Scott, Liz. "Why We Need Memoirs." *Millions*, July 1, 2019. https://themillions.com/2019/07/why-we-need-memoirs.html.

Sundberg, Kelly. "Can Confessional Writing Be Literary?" *Brevity* (blog), February 22, 2016. https://brevity.wordpress.com/tag/trauma-and-writing/.

Williams, Alison K. "Don't Be Brave." *Brevity* (blog), November 3, 2014. https://brevity.wordpress.com/2014/11/03/dont-be-brave/.

Books on the Craft of Memoir and Writing about Trauma

Baxter, Charles. *The Art of Subtext: Beyond Plot.*

Bell, Jerri, Carmelinda Blagg, and James Mathews. *Copy That! The Creative Writer's Military Style Guide.*

Capps, Ron. *Writing War: A Guide to Telling Your Own Story.*

Chee, Alexander. *How to Write an Autobiographical Novel.*

Crow, Tracy. *On Point: A Guide to Writing the Military Story.*

Goldberg, Natalie. *Writing Down the Bones: Freeing the Writer Within.*

Gornick, Vivian. *The Situation and the Story: The Art of Personal Narrative.*

Gutkind, Lee. *You Can't Make This Stuff Up: The Complete Guide to Writing Creative Nonfiction from Memoir to Literary Journalism and Everything in Between.*

Lamott, Ann. *Bird by Bird: Some Instructions on Writing and Life.*

Pennebaker, James W., and John F. Evans. *Expressive Writing: Words That Heal.*

Pennebaker, James W., and Joshua M. Smyth. *Opening Up by Writing It Down: How Expressive Writing Improves Health and Eases Emotional Pain.* 3rd ed.

Zinsser, William. *Writing about Your Life: A Journey into the Past.*

Books on Processing Trauma

Caruth, Cathy. *Unclaimed Experience: Trauma, Narrative, and History.* 20th anniversary ed.

Frankl, Viktor E. *Man's Search for Meaning.*

Herman, Judith Lewis. *Trauma and Recovery: The Aftermath of Violence—from Domestic Abuse to Political Terror.*

Marinella, Sandra. *The Story You Need to Tell: Writing to Heal from Trauma, Illness, or Loss.*

My Favorite Memoirs, Autobiographies, and Personal Essay Collections

Agassi, Andre. *Open: An Autobiography.*

Baldwin, James. *Notes of a Native Son.*

Barber, Charles. *Songs from the Black Chair.*

Broyard, Bliss. *One Drop: My Father's Hidden Life—a Story of Race and Family Secrets.*

Burroughs, Augusten. *Dry: A Memoir.*

———. *Running with Scissors.*

———. *A Wolf at the Table.*

Busch, Benjamin. *Dust to Dust: A Memoir.*

Caputo, Philip. *A Rumor of War.*

Carr, David. *The Night of the Gun: A Reporter Investigates the Darkest Story of His Life—His Own.*

Castner, Brian. *The Long Walk: A Story of War and the Life That Follows.*

Christman, Jill. *Dark Room.*

Coates, Ta-Nehisi. *Between the World and Me.*

Cowser, Bob. *Greenfields.*

Cranston, Bryan. *A Life in Parts.*

Dubus, Andre, III. *Townie: A Memoir.*

Finnegan, William. *Barbarian Days: A Surfing Life.*

Finneran, Kathleen. *The Tender Land: A Family Love Story.*

Friedman, Matti. *Pumpkin Flowers: A Soldier's Story.*

Fussel, Paul. *Doing Battle: The Making of a Skeptic.*

Gourevitch, Philip. *We Wish to Inform You That Tomorrow We Will Be Killed with Our Families: Stories from Rwanda.*

Grealy, Lucy. *Autobiography of a Face.*

Hainey, Michael. *After Visiting Friends: A Son's Story.*

Handler, Jessica. *Invisible Sisters.*

Hersh, Seymour M. *Reporter: A Memoir.*

Kalanithi, Paul. *When Breath Becomes Air.*

Karr, Mary. *Liar's Club.*

Kerman, Piper. *Orange Is the New Black: My Year in a Women's Prison.*

Kidder, Tracy. *My Detachment: A Memoir.*

King, Stephen. *On Writing: A Memoir of the Craft.*

Kingston, Maxine Hong. *The Woman Warrior.*

Kittredge, William. *A Hole in the Sky.*

Levy, Ariel. *The Rules Do Not Apply.*

Lowry, Beverly. *Crossed Over: A Murder, A Memoir.*

Manchester, William. *Goodbye, Darkness.*

Manguso, Sara. *The Two Kinds of Decay.*

Marlantes, Karl. *What It Is Like to Go to War.*

McInerny, Nora. *No Happy Endings: A Memoir.*

Mendelsohn, Daniel. *Lost: A Search for Six of Six Million.*

Nabokov, Vladimir. *Speak, Memory.*

Norman, Michael. *These Good Men: Friendships Forged from War.*

Orwell, George. *Homage to Catalonia.*

Sanders, Scott Russell. *The Paradise of Bombs.*

———. *A Private History of Awe.*

———. *Staying Put.*

Schwartz, Mimi. *Good Neighbors, Bad Times: Echoes of My Father's German Village.*

Sebald, W. G. *The Rings of Saturn.*

Sheff, David. *Beautiful Boy: A Father's Journey through His Son's Addiction.*

Sherman, Alexie. *You Don't Have to Say You Love Me.*

Slater, Lauren. *Welcome to My Country.*

Springsteen, Bruce. *Born to Run.*

Stack, Megan K. *Every Man in This Village Is a Liar: An Education in War.*

Strayed, Cheryl. *Wild: From Lost to Found on the Pacific Coast Trail.*

Stryon, William. *Darkness Visible.*

Trachtenberg, Peter. *The Book of Calamities.*

Tretheway, Natasha. *Beyond Katrina: A Meditation on the Mississippi Gulf Coast.*

Turner, Brian. *My Life as a Foreign Country: A Memoir.*

Walker, Jerald. *Street Shadows: A Memoir of Race, Rebellion, and Redemption.*

Walls, Jeannette. *The Glass Castle.*

Wamariya, Clementine, and Elizabeth Weil. *The Girl Who Smiled Beads.*

Wang, Esmé Weijun. *The Collected Schizophrenias.*

Ward, Jesmyn. *Men We Reaped.*

Wiesel, Elie. *Night.*

Wolff, Tobias. *This Boy's Life.*

David Chrisinger wears many hats as a writer and editor. He directs the Harris Writing Program at the University of Chicago, teaches writing seminars for The War Horse, and is a contributing writer for the *New York Times Magazine*'s At War column. His writing has also appeared in several other outlets, including *Collateral*; *War, Literature & the Arts*; *UChicago Magazine*; and *Reader's Digest*, as well as in several edited anthologies.

For three years, he taught a first-of-its-kind writing seminar for student veterans at the University of Wisconsin–Stevens Point, and in 2017, he wrote an instructor's manual for his class that is now available for adoption at every campus in the University of Wisconsin system. In 2016, David edited a collection of his students' essays titled *See Me for Who I Am* that is helping bridge the cultural gap dividing post-9/11 veterans from those who have not served.

For six years, David also taught public policy writing in the Master of Public Policy Program at the Bloomberg School of Public Health at Johns Hopkins University. In 2017, he wrote *Public Policy Writing That Matters*, a book for anyone passionate about using writing to create real and lasting policy change. The second edition is due out in 2022.

David is also writing a book for Penguin Press on Ernie Pyle, the famed World War II correspondent who followed front-line troops from North Africa to Italy, in France, and in the Pacific.

conflict: in achieving object of desire, 41–42; escalation, 113; as growth and transformation cause, 19–20, 54

confusion, 27, 157

connection, 140; through confidential stories, 188; between teacher and students, 184–85, 190–91; between writer and readers, 42–43, 179, 182–92

control, lack of, 40

coronavirus pandemic, 9

Costner, Kevin, 85

courage, 55, 139, 157, 191, 193

crime stories, 41

crises, 107, 109, 119, 123, 198

crying, 25, 44–45, 52–53, 166, 189, 198–99

Culman, Irene Stokes, 166–67

Damascus, Syria, 145–46, 148

dead bodies/body parts, exposure to, 9; of deceased loved ones, 35–37, 50, 52–53; in military combat, 21, 22, 23–25, 175, 178–79; relationship to the living person, 52–53

death: of children, 35–37, 39–40, 42–43, 61; exposure to, 9–10; fear of, 92–93; of grandparents, 49–53, 126, 140, 163–64; images associated with, 153–54; of parents, 51–52, 54, 61, 163–64

decision-making, 41–42; during climax, 119; during crisis, 119; in degeneration stories, 58; radical, 56; in revelation stories, 58

defensiveness, 183–84, 185–86

degeneration stories, 58

dénouement, 107

depression, 9, 21, 22, 57, 111, 166

description, 121–22; of characters, 88–91, 152

despair, 37, 111, 123

details, immersive, 149–55, 189

Diagnostic and Statistical Manual of Mental Disorders, fifth ed., 9

dialogue, speculative or imaginative, 179–80

Disappointment River: Finding and Losing the Northwest Passage (Castner), 80–81

disillusionment stories, 57–58

Dispatches (Herr), 87, 105–6

divorce, 69–70, 166, 195

domestic abuse, 61–62, 161–62, 172–73, 174

dramatic arc, 107

duty, 39, 55

Ebola virus, 9

editors, 87

education stories, 56–57

embarrassment, 46, 65, 87, 191

emotional core, 110

emotional expression, 44–45

empathy, 63, 65–66, 114, 176

endings, of stories, 39, 120–21; happy, 120, 194, 195, 199. See also resolution

endurance racing, 28, 30–34

EOD (explosive ordnance disposal) officers, 76–77

existence, reason for, 8

exposition, 109, 110

expressive writing, 5; difficulty with, 10–12; readiness for, 11–12; style, 6

Facebook, 6, 20, 21, 91, 92, 184

facts, relationship to truth, 172

failure, dealing with, 182–88

faith, in oneself and others, 55

family stories, untold, 44–45, 50, 53, 54

fatal flaws, in literature, 92–94

father-son relationships, 85–86, 162–63; changes over time, 55–56; estrangement in, 92

father-son relationship stories, 44–53, 54; characterization in, 67–73; as revelation stories, 58–66, 85–87

horror stories, 41
humanitarianism, 27–28
Hurt Locker, The (film), 76
Hussein, Saddam, 95, 96
hypervigilance, 26

ideals, 57
IEDs (improvised explosive devices), 3, 19, 23–25
imagination, 156, 159–60, 179–80
immersive scenes, 145–55
Immigration and Nationality Act, 145
inciting events, 108–13
industrial trauma, 10
infants, death of, 35–37, 39–41, 42–43
in medias res, 110
intergenerational trauma, 44–53
intimacy, 52, 174, 177
intrusive memories, 21, 22, 26
invulnerability, 42
Iowa State University, 145
Iraq, US invasion, 95–98
Iraqi refugees, 147
Iraq War veterans, 26, 28, 38, 76, 81–83
Iwo Jima, Battle of, 169

Jones, Edgar L., 169–70
Junger, Sebastian, 135

Kakazu Ridge, Okinawa, 126–30, 137
Kelly, Jack, 171
Kenosha, WI, 58, 68, 69
Kilpatrick, Dean G., 9

Ladies' Home Journal, 166
language: defensive, 183–84; descriptive, 105–6; figurative, 151–52
Letscher, Jack, 85, 127–30, 170–72
Letts, Tracy, 195
Library of Congress, Veterans History Project, 3, 5–6
life-threatening illnesses, 67–68

listening, supportive, 23, 191
Long Walk, The (Castner), 81–83, 87
loss, 27, 120; disillusionment over, 57–58, 59; ennobling nature of, 57; of family members, 9; fear of, 92–93; of friends, 108–9; of goals, 58; of infants and children, 35–41, 42–43; transformative nature of, 28–29
love, 55; expression of, 69
love stories, 41
lying, 156–57

Mackenzie, Alexander, 71
Mackenzie River canoe trip, 71–81, 83–92
Madison, WI, 96
main character, 41, 54; decision-making, 41–42; in degeneration stories, 58; in disillusionment stories, 57–58; in education stories, 56–57; at end of story, 120; goals of, 56; in maturing stories, 56–57; of memoirs, 195–96; personal growth, 56–57; in revelation stories, 58
Manchester, William, 134–35
Man's Search for Meaning (Frankl), 7, 8
Marine Corps, 6, 22, 94–97; war atrocities, 169; in WWII, 168–69
Marine Corps veterans: confessional/confidential stories, 182–89; sense of purpose, 27, 28. *See also* Afghan War veterans; Foley, Brett
Marquette University, 76
maturing stories, 56, 57–58
McLean, Kate, 106
meaningfulness, 57, 113, 116; restoration of, 22–23
meaningful relationships, 29, 30
medical professionals, coronavirus pandemic–related trauma, 9
melancholy, 37–38